The Weight-Loss Prescription

The Weight-Loss Prescription

A Doctor's Plan for Permanent Weight Reduction and Better Health for Life

Ali Zentner, MD

PENGUIN
an imprint of Penguin Canada

Published by the Penguin Group
Penguin Group (Canada), 90 Eglinton Avenue East, Suite 700, Toronto, Ontario, Canada M4P 2Y3

Penguin Group (USA) Inc., 375 Hudson Street, New York, New York 10014, U.S.A.
Penguin Books Ltd, 80 Strand, London WC2R 0RL, England
Penguin Ireland, 25 St Stephen's Green, Dublin 2, Ireland (a division of Penguin Books Ltd)
Penguin Group (Australia), 707 Collins Street, Melbourne, Victoria 3008, Australia
(a division of Pearson Australia Group Pty Ltd)
Penguin Books India Pvt Ltd, 11 Community Centre, Panchsheel Park, New Delhi – 110 017, India
Penguin Group (NZ), 67 Apollo Drive, Rosedale, Auckland 0632, New Zealand
(a division of Pearson New Zealand Ltd)
Penguin Books (South Africa) (Pty) Ltd, 24 Sturdee Avenue, Rosebank, Johannesburg 2196, South Africa

Penguin Books Ltd, Registered Offices: 80 Strand, London WC2R 0RL, England

First published 2013

2 3 4 5 6 7 8 9 10 (WEB)

Manufactured in Canada.

LIBRARY AND ARCHIVES CANADA CATALOGUING IN PUBLICATION

Zentner, Ali
The weight-loss prescription : a doctor's plan for permanent weight reduction and better health for life / Ali Zentner.

Includes index.

ISBN 978-0-14-318767-7

1. Reducing diets. 2. Weight loss. I. Title.

RM222.2.Z46 2013 613.2'5 C2012-905155-1

Contents

For my patients who make it a joy and not a job.
For Jason who makes it a life.

Author's Note

The accounts of the patients highlighted in this book are all real. Their permission was sought, of course, before using their stories, and their names and certain details of their lives have been changed to preserve their privacy.

My husband was not so lucky; he does indeed think chocolate milk is healthy but will now likely never drink it again.

Dr. Harvey Rabin is also real. He is a legend and a fabulous human being—the world should know his name.

Introduction

We have heard all too often about the scope of the problem. It's on every television, in every magazine, and has been the topic of countless books. Libraries across North America are filled with pages detailing just how bad obesity has become. We call it an epidemic of "mass proportions"; we make witty plays using the *f* word; we talk about "the weight of the matter" and how we're in "big trouble."

Maybe it's time for a change in perspective. If knowledge really is power, and an attitude can save this broken world, then maybe we have more to learn than we realize.

I spend my days in perpetual learning. I am surrounded by some of the bravest and most inspiring people this country has to offer. They are my patients, and they fight the disease known as obesity. I want their stories to be a lesson in compassion; I want my experiences with them to be a journey to the science of this disease.

I can no longer tolerate the mainstream message suggesting that losing weight is an impossibility and that behaviours cannot be changed. I have seen firsthand what behavioural psychology has spent decades screaming from the towers—people *can* change, and people *want* to change. More importantly, they want to be inspired to do so. Let this be the book that inspires people to look at weight loss in a dramatically different way. Let this be more than just lessons learned—let this be the place to begin.

I'm not naïve. I know that this will not be the last weight-loss book you ever read. Obesity is a disease that is ever-changing, and we are learning more about it each day. Our world is constantly evolving and this area of medicine will change with it. So, no, this is not the *last diet book* you'll ever look at. Instead, this is likely the first book that says "*I know you can*" and gives you the tools for a true lifestyle change.

Let's be frank—diets don't work. By their nature, they are only for a fixed period in time. They operate based on the principle that people need to suffer, restrict, deny, and deceive but *only* for a fixed period of time. Diets offer a beginning, middle, and an end.

Lifestyle changes, however, offer a completely different mindset and a way of doing things. So let's try a different way of doing things: Let's try *not* to diet. Let's try a big bold lifestyle change, but let's try it one step at a time.

A lifestyle change is more than just words. I know many people think it is just "semantics." They think calling something a "diet" or a "lifestyle change" is just talk. But language is important. I'll state my bias here: I'm a fan of words. Words diagnose, they treat, and they heal. In my daily practice, a world where treatment options for obesity are at best limited, all we have are the words we choose to hear and the ones we tell ourselves. And in those words there is the key.

I know what you're thinking: "Who does she think she is? What does she know about weight loss? What does she know about obese people?" The answer is *a lot.* I've spent the last decade treating patients of all sizes and risks ("in the trenches," so to speak). I've devoted my career to understanding what makes a person obese and how to treat the disease. I've committed all of my training and education to understanding the relatively new science emerging on an ancient disease.

But more importantly, I was my first patient. I'm not *just* an obesity doctor—I'm an obesity survivor. In 2000 I weighed 322 pounds; when I weighed myself this morning the scale read 148. Sure it was first thing in the morning and I was naked, but that is definitely more than just water weight. It's safe to say that I've been there—in mind, body, and practice.

There is more to this, however, than just the pounds I have lost or the patients I have seen. If I had to keep count, I would estimate that I've had the honour of treating over 5000 patients specifically for obesity over the past decade. I am not successful with all of them, but fortunately, life and medicine do not keep score. It's not so much about the number of pounds lost in practice or in theory; rather, in obesity medicine, it is about the message that is sent. I would like to think each patient leaves my office better off than when he or she arrived.

I sit in my office each day and listen. I listen to patients pour out their hearts—some with tears, some with anger and frustration. I see them feel hope and despair. Their stories about their struggles are varied yet often similar. I often think about the lessons they have to teach. Their stories inspire me to improve my own health and to continue on with other patients.

The magnitude of the effect is difficult to measure, though. For example, how do you measure the effect you have on someone's life? How do you quantify your contribution to another individual's day? Is my effect as an obesity physician purely a function of how much weight each of my patients loses? Or do we need to think beyond that for a moment? There has to be a message behind the hundreds of thousands of visits and the lives spent fighting this disease. A story must inspire, but it also must inform. The information must then be used to effect change. And now it is time to share what I know and what I have learned with other patients like mine and other people like me ... one step at a time.

Here's the interesting thing: We have rules that govern every part of our lives. We have rules of conduct regarding how we will let other people treat us and how we will act in kind. We have rules about how we allow others to speak to us and spend time with us. We have a code of conduct that designates our daily behaviour. We *do not*, however, have rules regarding one of the most important relationships in our lives—the one we have with food. I see it every day in the patients I treat and the people I meet. We have let mainstream culture dictate our code of conduct for our relationship with food. Media, advertising, and mainstream culture have been allowed to run amok and make our rules for us.

What if we set forth with a new set of rules? A positive set of rules—ones that were proactive and helped us transform our future health. I am not interested in a negative connotation here: I want these rules to be a positive code of conduct that governs our behaviour in such a way as to guide us how to be healthy—a compassionate set of do's and don'ts, if you will. Human beings have evolved over hundreds of thousands of years to store fat. As a species we are pretty great at *not* starving to death, even in times of famine. As a member of the medical community I am often shocked at the lack of advanced therapies in place for a disease as prevalent as obesity. Why have we left it to the mainstream to help us lose weight?

My ultimate question is this: How do we, in the absence of advanced therapies, alter our behaviour toward food? Can we establish certain patterns of behaviour that allow us to re-examine and then reshape our actions? I believe we can. In the first eight chapters of this book we will do just that—examine certain patterns of behaviour that each of us possesses toward food, and then put forth a plan for modifying these behavioural patterns.

Along the way I'll introduce you to various "Eating Personalities," which are personified by personal stories of patients I have treated over the years. These are classic patients whose patterns of behaviour act as a lesson to all of us, showing what we can do to alter our own environments to effect a healthy change. These are people you will be able to identify with—someone whose patterns of behaviour reflect your own. You may, in fact, be a combination of one or more of these Eating Personalities. Regardless of which personality you are, they will give you a frame of reference.

Within each of the Eating Personalities chapters I give you a place to begin for altering that behaviour. For example, are you an emotional eater? How do you know if you are? How do you engage in certain patterns of behaviour to control your emotional eating? Well, there's a chapter for you.

In Chapters 9 through 12, I will show you some general strategies to use that I call "a blueprint for change." I will give you techniques that I use in my everyday practice that are scientifically proven to help you change your relationship with food. I will show you how to keep a food diary and how to establish some positive food rules. Overall, I want you to create a kinder and more forgiving code of conduct for you and your relationship with food and your health.

Once we have a blueprint for change we will take a look at the road ahead. How do you take what you've learned about yourself and make some meaningful steps toward change? How do you evaluate where you are and where you realistically want to be? Is the change you are looking for a real possibility, or should you re-evaluate your goals and set some new ones? I will give you a glimpse into the world of positive psychology and show you some techniques for focusing on the here and now—how to live in the moment. Weight loss and lifestyle change is a lifelong process; how do you stay focused in the moment and not lose sight of your accomplishments?

In the final four chapters of this book, I'll outline how to maintain your new patterns of behaviour. What do you do under special circumstances that life almost always presents to you? How do you get back on track when you lose your way? How do we really make lifestyle changes go the distance? Finally, we'll end with some specific meal plans and recipes to get you started on your new road to health.

Why I Wrote This Book

I've struggled with being overweight for most of my life. I was the chubby kid in high school. I can remember my mother taking me to the first of many nutritionists at the age of nine—I weighed 120 pounds and the diet she put me on involved a lot of tuna. I guess I've spent three decades on one diet or another. My twenties were spent gaining and losing the same thirty or forty pounds over and over again. In medical school the work and the hours of sitting and studying took their toll on me, and I graduated with a degree and an extra thirty pounds. Residency was an all-time low point in my health and my struggle with obesity. I easily gained a hundred pounds. It was almost too easy to finish each night of being on call with chicken fingers, french fries, and a carton of Ben & Jerry's ice cream. If I wasn't at the hospital, I was on the couch eating ice cream.

I loved food. More importantly, I loved sugar. I ate ice cream by the carton and bags of Werther's caramels. I would bargain in my head that the caramels were only ten calories each, and that I was only eating ice cream for dinner and nothing else, so somehow it was justified. Furthermore, I hated exercise. First of all, it hurt. I was big and movement was not fun. Second, I somehow never had the time; days blended into each other. My clothes slowly stopped fitting and I would just buy a bigger size. Once the size eighteen suits did not fit, then came size twenty, twenty-two, and so on. It's as if I woke up one day four years into residency and I weighed 322 pounds. I almost don't remember how it happened, but I was seriously stuck.

And then one day I started to change. Make no mistake—it was not like I woke up one day and decided "today's the day." In fact, I would argue that I spent most of my adult life waking up with that sentiment in my mind. But if I had to think back to a specific point in my life where the crack first appeared in the ceiling, I would recall my thirtieth birthday, when I was in the last year of my residency. I made myself an entire pot of Kraft Dinner, sat down on the couch with a bottle of red wine, and cried. This was not the first time I had eaten an entire pot of pasta with alcohol and tears on board, but somehow, over a decade later, this day stands out in my memory. I was really miserable. My life was not where it should have been. Sure, from a career standpoint I had done pretty well for myself. I was, after all, on my way to being a specialist. I was happily married to a man who never said a word about the bags of candy around the house. He loved me—sweet tooth and all.

Despite my size and my headspace I somehow knew that my life had to have more than just this. I don't remember when or where it happened, but I recall this feeling that I could do something about it. I began to spend my time learning all I could about the physiology of obesity and about nutrition. In medicine we learn from each patient, because each patient teaches us something new about a disease. I *was* my first obesity patient; I used my own experiences as a framework for what to do and what to learn.

When I think about what I have accomplished since then, I see myself as part of a process. We all have a beginning and an end in life, but I feel the process of life is more than that. I've gone from crying on a couch with macaroni and cheese to running marathons. More importantly, I'm amazed at how far I've come. I am amazed at how my life continues to "open up" in a variety of ways. New sports, new opportunities ... there really do not seem to be any limitations.

Health is never the default. Health is the choice, the fight, and the active state. It's what we always have to work at. But when we come to that fight with a sense of positivity and a sense of who we are, we are never let down by our abilities.

I realize that my story is not the norm. Many patients will try but not reach their goals. What they need to know is that *tenacity* is the way to go—giving up is not an option. Once you figure out who you are there are no limits to your abilities. In life, we really are all superheroes—we just need to figure out what cape to wear.

The Weight-Loss Prescription

1

The Power of Food

Think about it for a minute … what other substance on the planet is good for you, is necessary for life, and is truly enjoyable? Nothing satisfies these three criteria except food.

I think this is likely the root of the problem when it comes to our relationship (healthy or not) with food. Food really is necessary for life. Our bodies have an intricate system of adaptation, developed over thousands of years, that is geared toward seeking out food, consuming it for immediate use for energy, or conserving it in the form of stored energy (or fat) for later.[1] Moreover, many foods aren't just necessary for life but are indeed good for you. Certain foods have been shown to improve our cardiovascular health; others have been linked to a reduction in the development of certain diseases; other components of food build healthier tissues and bodies.[2]

Finally, food is fun. Show me someone who does not enjoy the taste of a great piece of apple pie and I will show you someone who's just never had one. Food is so much a part of who we are as a society and how we express ourselves. We celebrate and we mourn through food. We express ourselves through how we prepare and consume food, and many of our societal and cultural norms revolve around how we eat and what we eat.

I'm no different than many obese people; my love of food started early. In 1980, when I was nine years old, my mother took me to my first nutritionist. Her name was Elizabeth. She was a lovely woman with a sweet voice and very short, curly hair. I was in Grade 3 and I weighed 120 pounds. If I close my eyes I can still see her office. It was on the tenth floor of an office building on a main street in Winnipeg with a window view of the legislature. I remember sitting in Elizabeth's office every Monday at 4 P.M., waiting to be weighed and measured. I spent much of Grade 3 and half of Grade 4 counting the seasons as they changed while watching the statue of the Golden Boy that sits atop the dome of the legislature.

At our first meeting, Elizabeth told me that if I stayed the same weight, by the age of twenty I would be just fine. She outlined a diet with a list of foods that I could and could not eat and put together a menu plan for me to follow. I remember there being a lot of milk and a lot of dry tuna with no mayonnaise. And so began my journey into the world of dieting.

Unfortunately, Elizabeth and I did not see eye to eye. Now I can see that she was trying her best, but it was the early 80s, after all, and when it came to managing kids with a weight problem the scientific community was really at a disadvantage. We knew very little about why some kids gained weight and others didn't. Elizabeth was just working with what she had at the time.

And I did not make it easy for Elizabeth. I remember going home from our Monday visits with my blank food diaries in my hand and chocolate cake on my brain. I could not wait to cheat on this diet. My mother, on the other hand, was excited and convinced that this would be the solution to my problems. On Tuesday mornings my mother began her mission. My school lunches were lovingly prepared the night before—dry tuna, carrot sticks, and a piece of fruit. I spent much of my grade school years unpacking my lunches with significant disappointment.

Janet was my best friend in Grade 3, and we were inseparable. We played together at recess and ate together at lunch. Janet weighed forty-five pounds. I know this because she once told me that in Grade 1 she weighed as much as a neighbour's cat. Janet was "petite," as her mother called her, and although we were inseparable, we could not have been more opposite when it came to appearances. If you stood us next to each other we looked like a caricature. I was round and average height and she was tiny and slender. Janet was the littlest girl in our class and I was the biggest in our school. When you put us together we looked like Laurel and Hardy. In fact, if memory serves me correctly, we even dressed up as them one year for Halloween. Upon reflection, my choice in best friend only reinforced my size. I don't blame Janet for being tiny any more than I blame myself for being big. It's just an interesting turn of events that the girl I spent most of my childhood with never had a weight problem in her life. Looking back, I can see all too well where my problems began.

The contrast between Janet and me only serves to highlight that I really do have a disease and Janet does not. But what fascinates me even further is how I built my world around food and kept my disease going. I learned a lot about normal food behaviours from Janet and my own lack of them. Being friends with her served to highlight what was wrong with me.

When we were nine years old, Janet and I spent a lot of time at the movies. We would get dropped off at the theatre for the Sunday matinee show and make a real event of it. I remember the first time our parents let us go to the movies by ourselves. I was given $5 for the day. The movie was $2.50 and the remaining money went to popcorn and licorice. I love licorice—to this day it is the taste of my childhood. I would buy the largest bag they had at the theatre and a large drink. Because I was a "fat kid" my mother had already conditioned me to only drink diet pop. I remember ripping into the licorice before we even reached our seats. I would use each sugary vine as a straw to sip the cold pop and then repeatedly, rhythmically, finish one licorice stick after another. I was in a sugar trance as I systematically went through the entire package.

My licorice was gone before the first coming attractions hit the screen. I looked over at Janet. My package of licorice was empty and her stash was almost untouched. She was easily still savouring her second or third piece, and then did something so foreign to me that it has been imprinted on my brain ever since. She folded up the package of licorice and put it into her Hello Kitty purse.

"What are you doing?" I asked, in a bit of shock.

"I'm saving it for later." she said.

"Oh." I sat there in silence. I was in awe and in horror. How could she save it for later? Was that even possible? Who does that? Would I ever be able to save anything for later? Absolutely not. First of all, I was nine years old. Most kids can't save sugary treats for later any more than a hedonist can save pleasure for later. Asking a kid to put away a chocolate bar and do something else is just ridiculous. But Janet could put away the licorice and watch the movie without a care in the world.

Needless to say I spent the remainder of that movie fixated on the licorice in Janet's purse. I couldn't even concentrate on the film because my brain was so focused on the candy. I know Janet sensed something was wrong, because halfway through the movie she turned to me and asked, "Are you okay?"

"No," I confessed.

"What's wrong?" she asked, concerned.

And I voiced the only thing I could think of that would end the madness and allow me to enjoy the afternoon: "Janet, can I have the rest of your licorice?"

Even before that day at the movie I knew I was different than the other kids. I looked different than most of the other kids, and my lunches were certainly different. No other kid had to leave school early on Mondays to go see a nutritionist. But it was in that movie theatre, with Janet's licorice talking to me from inside her Hello Kitty purse, that I realized I was really different. Food had a power over me unlike any other substance. Food owned me unlike it did other kids. The other kids in my class had peanut butter sandwiches and homemade chocolate chip cookies in their lunches. I could smell the differences from the minute I unhinged my Wonder Woman lunch box. They would eat their lunches, or they would not eat their lunches and could easily throw out the food they did not like or trade it with other kids. Food had a power over me that I could not explain. I thought about it all the time and I mapped my daily events and emotions based on what meal I was facing.

As I moved through my medical career, I learned the science behind what I had discovered in that movie theatre so many years ago: The brain of an obese person really is different.[3] Even more elaborate than that, like so many other diseases obesity has a genetic predisposition and complexity that has yet to be fully understood. There is a biochemistry and physiological basis for why some people sit in a movie theatre and have a mental conversation with a package of licorice and others just watch the movie.[4] Decades of scientific study into this disease have established that a person's relationship with food is in part genetically predetermined.[5] Furthermore, there is an intricate system in the body that is highly evolved to regulate body weight.

First of all, we know that "fatness" does in fact run in families. Body weight is as potently influenced by genetics as is body height. Over 450 genes have been isolated that are linked to obesity.[6] Most of these genes operate at various levels of heredity. A study published in the *Journal of the American Medical Association* in 1986 attempted to calculate the heritability of a variety of diseases and traits in the North American population.[7] "Heritability" is the proportion of a trait that could be attributable to genetics. For example, eye colour is almost a hundred percent genetically predetermined. Diseases, on the other hand, are subject to varying environmental influences. What is most surprising about this study was that it showed that the heritability of obesity in a person was higher than the heritability of breast cancer, hypertension, or heart disease.

An even more fascinating study on the genetics of this disease shows that appetite and cravings can also be inherited.[8] Let's take the FTO gene, for example. The FTO gene has not only been shown to be linked to obesity, but also to food choices and cravings. The FTO variant is common, especially among certain ethnocultural groups. Approximately 65 percent of people of both European and African descent carry the gene, as do 27–44 percent of people of Asian descent. Studies from the University of Exeter show that people who carry the FTO gene have a much higher risk of developing obesity. Because we inherit one set of chromosomes from each parent, we all have two copies of every gene in our body. For example, you will inherit one copy of the FTO gene from your mom and one copy of the FTO gene from your dad. Studies show that people with one copy of the FTO gene have a 30 percent increase in their risk for obesity, while those with two copies of the gene have a 60 percent increase in obesity risk.

The studies don't point to exactly how the FTO gene increases one's risk of weight gain, but one study of Scottish schoolchildren may shed some light on the situation.[9] In 2008, a group of one hundred Scottish schoolchildren participated in three separate observed eating studies. These kids were put into a room with a variety of snacks ranging from fruits and vegetables to chips and chocolate. Each child was closely monitored regarding his or her total amount of food consumed. All food was weighed and measured before the kids were allowed to eat it. At the end of the trial the amount of food eaten by each child was compared, as was the total calorie counts and nutritional content of the snacks consumed. Finally, saliva from each of the subjects was collected to see if the child carried the FTO gene. Sure enough, children with the FTO variant ate at least one hundred calories more than the non-FTO kids. Furthermore, kids with the FTO variant were far more likely to consume foods higher in fat and refined sugar. These results were reproduced on three separate occasions at three separate observed eating sessions. I often wonder how many of my patients (their doctor included) would prove to have copies of the FTO gene or others like it.

Genetics is only one part of a very complex puzzle, however. And, as I have learned from more than a decade in medicine, genetics is not destiny. Your biochemical code plays a role in how your body responds to the environment around it, but it does not determine that response entirely.

How Big Is the Problem?

I refer to obesity a lot in this book, even though many of my patients hate the word. In fact, a recent survey suggests that patients prefer to initiate discussions about weight loss without using the term "obesity." I struggled for many months trying to establish a better terminology when talking about weight issues and healthy living, but not for lack of trying I came up short. That being said, this book is geared toward anyone who would like a healthier relationship with food, not just people who have weight issues.

The issue is that obesity is, in fact, a disease. Perhaps it doesn't have the same impact as a name like "cancer" or the scientific connotations like "atherosclerosis," but it is a disease nonetheless. There is a genetic background to this illness, a physiological feedback mechanism, a target tissue of action, and a host of environmental triggers that all play a role in the development of what we call obesity. The problem is that obesity implies a host of judgments against one's character and personality. Just the word "obesity" or even "overweight" implies that the person with this condition lacks certain empirical character traits that would allow them to do something about their size.

Science has spent decades establishing that this rather closed-minded view could not be further from the truth.[10] That being said, we as a culture have a ways to go in recognizing this. I would argue that we are with obesity in 2013 where we were with depression in the 1960s. In the 1960s, if a woman was diagnosed with depression she would never admit it in social circles. She might whisper it to her friend over coffee, if she were so brave. She was under the social impression that having depression was a fault in her character and her ability to just "snap out of it." And if she did reveal her condition to others, she was likely to be subjected to social scrutiny and alienation. I can't help but see the comparison today with many of my patients. Furthermore, obese individuals cannot hide their condition from others, as you can with some other diseases. As such, when it comes to judgment and ridicule it is often open season.

That being said, I have always maintained that when you give something a name you give it a voice. A name confers power and legitimacy on people and things—even diseases. Sometimes in my practice I see people for whom there is no diagnosis for their cluster of symptoms. Their common response is, "I just wish I had a diagnosis." So until we can come up with a different name, let's call this disease of the brain, belly, and body what it is—being overweight and obese. If you are obese or overweight and hate those terms, I suggest that you try not to get caught up in the label or the name. Instead, focus your energies on the fact that this is a disease and use its name as a platform to reclaim the empathy from a society that is deservedly yours.

The Weight of the World

The most interesting thing to me about obesity is that it is a disease that can be diagnosed just by looking at someone. Walk outside and look around—you can easily see how many people in your city or town are affected by this disease. You can tell, more often than not, by looking at someone whether they have a weight problem. But make no mistake—it is not actually that simple. Many obese people lead very healthy lives, and many non-obese people suffer from hypertension, diabetes, and heart disease. But you can't ignore the strong correlation between excess weight and certain diseases.

In 2001, I became a fully licensed specialist in internal medicine. My parents flew with me to Ottawa for the ceremony where I would officially become a specialist. I walked across a huge stage and bowed before the registrar to be "hooded" as a Fellow of the Royal College of Physicians and Surgeons of Canada. In that same year, less than 20 percent of Canadians and less than 25 percent of Americans were obese.

By the time this book reaches bookshelves that number will have more than doubled.

According to the 2009 Canadian Community Health Survey, 56.6 percent of Canadians aged 18 or older were considered overweight or obese. This translates into an estimated 12.6 million adults with a body mass index (BMI) of 25 or more. More than 60 percent of Americans fall into this same category. I would argue that the prevalence of obesity in North America translates into the greatest public health crisis this continent has ever seen.

But never mind statistics. Go outside into your city or town and look around—you don't have to be a doctor to see what is happening all around us. Our countries and our communities are growing. I'm not talking about bigger populations—I'm talking about a bigger collective body mass index.

Adolphe Quetelet first established the body mass index, or BMI, in the 1840s when he was trying to develop the concept of "social physics."[11] It was first named the Quetelet Index and was calculated by dividing a person's weight in kilograms by their height in metres to the power of two:

$$\text{BMI} = \text{Weight (kg)} / \text{Height (m)}^2$$

BMI first became popular in the early 1950s when Metropolitan Life Insurance Company used it as a means of determining risk for its future customers.[12] As the calculation implies, BMI does not measure percentage of body fat. In 1972, Dr. Ancel Keys, considered the father of modern-day cholesterol medicine, first looked at the correlation of BMI and cardiovascular risk.[13] Since then BMI has been widely used as a means of determining risk.

Unfortunately, like many risk calculators, the body mass index is not a perfect system.[14] It does not always correlate with risk; for example, a patient who is overweight or obese may in fact be at lower risk for heart disease than a much thinner counterpart when other risk factors are taken into account.

So what's the take-home message? BMI is not the only way to determine a person's health. Rather, it is a piece of the puzzle and must be evaluated in the context of a person's other risk factors such as other illnesses and family history.

I was the biggest kid in all of my grade school classes. Elizabeth tried her best, but she was up against a force of such intensity that I believe she was ill equipped to really help me. That was thirty years ago. Elementary school classes look much different today than they did three decades ago, especially when you look at children's weight. In fact, data from the Harvard School of Public Health shows that almost 25 percent of children under a year of age are clinically obese.[15] Obesity has reached epidemic proportions. If I found myself back in Grade 4 today, I suspect I would be one of many obese children. Ironically, I bet I would have as many options for weight loss as I had thirty years ago.

My father wanted me to be a doctor more than anything else in the world. My father was also the first person to take me to a Weight Watchers meeting. I was eleven years old and we got special permission from my pediatrician to attend. We would go to weigh-ins on Thursday nights, and then he would take me out for ice cream. My father was clinically obese. I think it was one of the things that bonded us from the beginning. Much of my relationship with food I learned from my dad. It is interesting to me that I went into medicine for my dad, and even more fascinating that I chose an area of medicine that would have undoubtedly made him my patient.

At the time that I got my degree I knew I wanted to do internal medicine as a specialty, but I had only a vague idea of what area of internal medicine would be my subspecialty. I knew I wanted to treat people with complex medical issues, and I knew I wanted to focus on areas of medicine that involved chronic disease. But my ambitions ended there. I think back to how much has changed since my parents attended that formal ceremony in Ottawa and watched me receive my official fellowship from the Royal College of Physicians and Surgeons. I watched my dad crying like a schoolchild and wondered where this profession would take me.

I moved to a small town in southern Alberta and began a practice in internal medicine. I treated patients with diabetes, hypertension, heart disease, and cancer. Patients were sent to me when they had a disease that was difficult to diagnose or when they had a medical problem that was difficult to manage. I spent the first six months of my practice doing the usual things doctors do—it was a pretty predictable practice for a specialist.

And then Bonnie walked into my office. Bonnie was thirty-seven years old the first time I saw her, and she was easily a hundred pounds overweight. She had gestational diabetes during all of her pregnancies, and she was referred to me for increasing fatigue. I took a detailed history from Bonnie and found out that she had been increasingly thirsty over the last few months. She was also noticing that she was having to urinate much more frequently. Bonnie had classic symptoms of hyperglycemia (elevated blood sugar) in keeping with new onset type 2 diabetes.

Type 2 diabetes is caused by a completely different mechanism than type 1 diabetes. Type 1 diabetes is an autoimmune disorder where the body's immune system attacks the insulin-producing cells in the pancreas know as beta cells. As a result, the beta cells are killed off and the body no longer produces insulin.[16] Insulin is how the body uses sugar as an energy source. Every cell, particularly our brain cells, needs insulin to function. Insulin binds to receptors on the cell surface to allow sugar to enter a cell and be used for energy. Without insulin, the cell can't use sugar as an energy source.

Type 2 diabetes is a whole different disease mechanism. Not only is there no lack of insulin (particularly in the beginning phases of the disease), but there is actually an abundance of insulin. With type 2 diabetes the difference is that there is a degree of insulin resistance. This means that the body's insulin cell receptors are not working properly and insulin does not bind properly to the receptors. In response, the body actually thinks that there is not enough insulin around and signals the pancreas to produce more insulin.[17] As a result, people in the beginning phases of type 2 diabetes have insulin resistance, not insulin deficiency.

Obesity is strongly linked to insulin resistance.[18] Fat cells themselves produce a variety of hormones that trigger insulin resistance, which is why obesity is such a strong risk factor for the development of type 2 diabetes. This is also why weight loss is such a powerful tool in the prevention and treatment of type 2 diabetes. When you lose weight, you shrink your fat cells. This decreases their hormonal activity and in turn shuts off the hormones that contribute to insulin resistance. As a result, you make the body more sensitive to insulin. If you are a type 2 diabetic with insulin resistance, you can see how important improving insulin resistance would be in treating your disease in the first place.

And so Bonnie walked into my office. I diagnosed her almost immediately with type 2 diabetes based on her risk factors (meaning her weight and her history of diabetes during pregnancy) and her symptoms. I had a blood glucometer in my office that I used to check patients' blood glucose levels, and sure enough when I tested Bonnie her numbers were off the charts.

There she was—thirty-seven years of age and a new diabetic. She began to cry. I did the usual things that I had learned to do over the years. Remember, I was relatively new to practice but I still knew all too well how to break bad news to people. I consoled Bonnie and gave her the requisite tissues. And then she said something that has stuck with me to this day. She uttered the most common sentence I hear when I diagnose an obese person with diabetes:

"I can't believe I let this happen to myself. How could I have let this happen?"

My heart sank. I was relatively new to obesity medicine, but even then I knew that Bonnie's weight was more than just a function of her will to let things happen. After all, I had spent years asking myself the same question. You see, as doctors we are sometimes taught that we are not supposed to identify with patients on a personal level. Our ability to be objective in a clinical situation is often crucial to our ability to make important decisions. At least that is how I used to feel. My ability to empathize with my patients continues to be one of my greatest clinical strengths. I no longer see objectivity and detachment as one and the same in medicine. Instead, I have learned through more than a decade in this profession that one's personality can indeed be the greatest therapeutic tool a doctor can have—particularly in the field of obesity medicine.

And so where Bonnie was concerned, I committed the greatest clinical transgression I could—I saw myself in her. I *was* Bonnie; or rather, she was me in a few years' time. By the same token, in helping her I realized that I would indeed help myself.

Through the course of our visit she said to me, "Losing weight is really hard, Dr. Zentner, you know?" I certainly did. Like every obese patient in the country, I could not hide my disease from others. My patients knew I was obese. What they did not know at the time was that I had decided to do something about it. Sure, I could identify with Bonnie and I would argue that being obese probably helped me be a better doctor to her. But what Bonnie did not know was that six months prior to our visit I had embarked on a lifelong journey to be an example for my patients.

Make no mistake—at the time I really had no idea what I was doing. I had no grand vision for a healthier life or for being a better example to my patients. Instead, my road to health began quite honestly by chance. Shortly before I first met Bonnie I had pre-diabetes, high blood pressure, and was in the worst shape of my life. I was thirty-one years old and had the cardiac risk profile of someone twice my age. As all good stories go, mine began by chance. I had bought a lottery ticket in the hospital home lottery. Hospitals commonly have an annual lottery to raise funds, and on this occasion I decided that I was feeling lucky. I dreamed of winning the house or the car or an extravagant trip. Sure enough three weeks later an enthusiastic voice on the other end of the phone announced that I was the proud winner of … an elliptical trainer.

In retrospect that lottery changed my life. At the time, however, I really wanted to win the car. The elliptical and I did not have an immediate love affair. Like most home exercise equipment, I used mine for the first month to dry laundry. But one day I was going through my closet and I came upon my wedding dress. I was easily a hundred pounds heavier than I had been at our wedding, but for some reason I thought I might try the dress on. I could barely get it past my shoulders and I began to sob.

There it was: a picture of desperation and comedy. Me, sitting in our apartment in Calgary with a massive white meringue of a wedding dress around my hips sobbing in front of an elliptical trainer covered in wet underwear. The story had always been the same in the past. I had always gotten angry and fed up and tried to make a change in my dieting life and fallen off track and reverted to normal. But for some reason, this time, the story ended differently.

I took off the ill-fitting wedding dress and got on the elliptical trainer. Five minutes later I thought I was dying. My legs were burning, I was sweating up a storm, and I was panting. But the next day, I went back. And the next, and so on. Five minutes became ten, and then thirty, and before I knew it I was doing sixty minutes a day on that elliptical trainer. Two weeks into my elliptical experience, I started keeping a food diary. I looked at what I was eating and started to make slow deliberate changes. We no longer ordered Chinese food twice a week and I stopped eating candies by the bagful. Dinners were punctuated by pieces of fruit and not cartons of ice cream. Within six months I had lost forty pounds.

And so this takes me back to my visit with Bonnie. It dawned on me in those moments that I could help her. If I could start on a path to health, so could she. And so Bonnie and I sat together and mapped out a list of things for her to do—a place to start. In reality I gave Bonnie her first set of food rules. I took out a piece of paper and wrote down three things for her to do that month:

1. Go for a walk every day for at least fifteen minutes.
2. Keep a food diary: Write down everything you eat on a piece of paper and bring it to your next visit.
3. Stop drinking any sugary drinks, fruit juice, or pop.

Bonnie returned the next month and every month after that for almost three years. In that time she lost over sixty pounds. She no longer needed medications for her diabetes, and she became an avid walker and cyclist who did some sort of activity every day for an hour. When I left Lethbridge to move to Vancouver, Bonnie and I met for one last visit. She had decided to continue to see her family doctor every couple of months for weight-loss counselling and was going to join Weight Watchers for the ongoing weekly accountability she felt she needed. At our last visit, Bonnie handed me an envelope. In it was a beautiful card of thanks and the torn and tattered sheet of paper I had given her at our first visit with her first list of "rules."

"Take it," she said confidently, "I don't need it anymore."

To this day it is the best gift any patient has ever given me.

Bonnie was my first of many patients who have such a story; people who make small changes and wind up in a totally different place. In my three years in Alberta I treated over 1000 patients for obesity with talk and behavioural change. The medical community calls it "behavioural modification." Really, it's just about doing something different today, then again tomorrow, and making it stick.

In the three years I spent as Bonnie's doctor I, too, was a model patient. I lost an additional eighty pounds for a grand total of

120 pounds. Bonnie and I came from similar beginnings and wound up being role models for each other. It is therefore no surprise that studies show that physicians' attitudes toward their own weight significantly impact their discussions around weight loss with their patients.[19]

Let's be clear, Bonnie's predicament and mine were more than just the environment we found ourselves in. As you will read more about in the next chapter, science has established that there are intricate neuro-hormonal, biochemical, and physiological factors that regulate our response to food. However, we have created an environment that, for lack of a better word, is truly toxic. What we've done is create a lifestyle that challenges our genetic predispositions. Our bodies were never made for the environment we are currently living in. We have structured a society around an abundance of high-calorie, nutrient-poor foods that human beings were never built to handle. It can therefore be no surprise as to how fast obesity numbers are rising in North America given the environment we find ourselves in.

What would happen if we took a group of people who were lifelong non-smokers and locked them in a room filled with cigarette smoke? We would effectively force them to live in an environment that preselected who among them was genetically at risk for developing lung cancer. North America today is such an environment when it comes to food. We have created a society where high-calorie, processed foods are the standard. Coupled with that, we have systematically engineered activity out of our daily routine. It's no surprise, therefore, that we have challenged a physiology that is completely ill equipped for our modern-day challenges. Sure, maybe some of us have thriftier genes than others that allow us to better handle the myriad food commercials, food cues, and food culture at every turn, but the majority of us aren't so lucky.

When was the last time you saw an advertisement for a food product? Was it on television, in a magazine, or on a billboard?

Either way, we are constantly surrounded by an onslaught of food cues. Spend an hour of your day counting how many times you see some sort of advertisement for food or drink, then add in the number of times you pass by a restaurant or takeout place and you will come up with a number that is easily between forty and fifty instances.

According to the Media Dynamics publication *Media Matters*, a typical adult has a potential daily exposure to about 600 to 625 advertisements in any form.[20] About 270 of these exposures come from the major traditional media (TV, radio, magazines, and newspapers). The data further suggest that more than half of these advertisements are for food or beverages. That works out to more than 300 food cues per day!

A 2009 study published in *Health Psychology* out of Yale University took two groups of children and examined their food intake based on their exposure to food advertisements.[21] The study randomly separated elementary school children into two groups. One group was assigned to watch a cartoon that included food advertising, while the other group was assigned to watch a cartoon with non-food-related advertising. Both groups of kids were given a snack to eat while watching the cartoon. The group watching the cartoons with food advertisements ate 48 percent more snack than the group whose cartoon did not include food advertisements.

Maybe I do have the FTO gene or a similar variant, and undoubtedly I come from good overweight genetics. My father was certainly obese and had a love for food that rivalled my own. I am told that my grandmother was also a very big woman. On the other hand, I also spent a lot of time watching television as a kid, and I grew up in a world that, even back in the 70s, had plenty of food cues. Both back then and today, I live in a world that reminds me daily how good that movie theatre licorice really is.

Often when I am in my office with a patient I think back to those days with Elizabeth and her attempts to help me lose weight.

Did she have any idea how complex this disease really is? Did she really understand what she was up against? I think of how far obesity medicine has come in the last thirty years, and how far we have yet to go.

I'm often asked if I know what it takes to make a healthier community. The easy answer is that we need to return to an environment that respects what our bodies were meant to handle in terms of food. That would be great, but it would require that we all get together and change our social infrastructure to go back to the days when we physically worked hard for our food and our choices were guided more by nutrition and less by convenience and pleasure, and that's not realistic. People will not give up their cars en masse, and fast-food restaurants are here to stay. I am not being pessimistic, just realistic as to what we can expect from the world around us. The point is that we don't need that radical social restructuring to change our fate as a community. A healthier community is composed of healthier members, so instead let's talk about small steps that individuals can take to reshape their present and significantly impact their future.

Sure, you have a complex biochemistry that fights you at every turn and an environment that certainly does not help the situation. But in medicine as in life, we take what we are given and we make the best of things. Maybe you won't change the world, but you will create a revolution in your own life that will impact how you look at your health, yourself, and others. Now let's get started.

2

You Are How You Eat

Most of us think we know what the problem is when it comes to obesity and weight loss: We think it's simply that we don't exercise enough or we eat too much. Right now you are probably thinking about which group you fall into. Do I eat too much, or do I not exercise enough? Or is it both? Interestingly, you are wrong on both counts. Obesity is not a simple problem. Sure, most of us eat too much and don't move enough, but the physiology of this disease is so much more than one or even both of those concepts. But this is not a book about the physiology of the disease; this is a book about making behavioural changes for the better.

When the body loses weight, the brain tends to follow. Remember: We were designed to conserve fat. It is a biological and evolutionary survival skill so that primitive man could survive in periods of famine. The issue is that when we begin to restrict calories in any way, our brain actually becomes heightened toward this.[22] The hunger you feel when you change your eating habits is an SOS response that your brain sends out to your body to stay alive. After you've lost weight, areas of your brain that are involved in the emotional involvement of food and decision making are heightened—you lose emotional and cognitive-planning control, so you have less restraint over and less awareness of what you eat.

There is a significant satiation deficiency—your desire to eat is up and your inhibition to stop is down.[23] This is very much hard-wired into our physiology to ensure survival. The science of it all continues to amaze me and only reinforces how hard it can be to lose weight. However, I don't tell you this so that you will be disenchanted or disheartened. I don't want you to be discouraged by your physiology in any way.

So, because we can't alter our physiology, we have to alter our environment.

As you will see as you read this book and as you have seen throughout the course of your own life, losing weight is a constant battle. Here's the real challenge with any weight-loss program or any lifestyle change: We set goals we can never achieve. But what if we matched the complexity of a program with the capacity of the person to change? What if we set ourselves up for success by creating a program based on exactly what we are able to do? More importantly—what if we lived instead in the *now* and no longer focused on a long-term goal? I've long maintained that we should match our capacity for this process to its complexity. You may first ask yourself, "What is my capacity? What am I capable of?" Interestingly, I think that is what changes over time. A more important question to ask yourself is, "What is the complexity of the situation? How rigid are my surroundings when it comes to weight loss?"

We live in a world where food is a significant part of our culture. For most North Americans, food is how we celebrate and sometimes how we cope. Food is in part a window through which we communicate with the world. It is often how we show love, gratitude, and even remorse. I am not suggesting that we abandon our cultural norms when it comes to food, but I do think when those norms become abnormal there needs to be an adjustment in behaviour. If, for example, the only way I know how to say thank you is by baking three dozen cookies and eating half of them, then I have to find a healthier way to express my gratitude. This might seem extreme, but it illustrates my point.

So how do you look at your patterns of behaviour in a meaningful way and analyze them objectively? Most of us find it hard to figure out where we are going wrong. Human beings learn by mistake; unfortunately, we are so intolerant of these errors as a species that we often don't allow the lessons to be learned.

To help overcome this problem, I've established a set of "Eating Personalities." These are clear patterns of behaviour modelled after one or more of my patients that many people will be able to identify with. Regardless of how maladjusted your eating behaviours are, I suspect you may find yourself in at least one or more of these models of behaviour. Every one of us is one form of an overeating stereotype or another. Let's break it down to some simple concepts that every one of us can work through. More importantly, let's establish some parameters of new behaviour within these stereotypes so that we can change how we behave toward food.

In the pages that follow, I provide a brief description of each type. Then, in the next six chapters, I go into detail about how to "diagnose" yourself with each model and then, of course, how to do something about it. Remember, you have to do more than just find out *who* you are. You have to then translate that into some code of conduct. You have to establish some food rules and change your pattern of behaviour. I want you to look at who you are and how you behave around food and then restructure that behaviour in a stepwise process.

Let's get started. Remember that you may fall into one or more of these patterns of behaviour, so it's important to keep an open mind. The six Eating Personalities are as follows:

1. The emotional eater
2. The calorie drinker
3. The fast-food junkie
4. The all-or-nothing dieter
5. The portion distorter
6. The sitting duck

The Emotional Eater

The emotional eater is a person who uses food to meet some sort of emotional need. Emotional eaters use food as a crutch to help them get through times of sadness, stress, loneliness, or depression. Emotional eaters also use food in times of joy or as reward. There are even emotional eaters who use food as an activity in times of boredom.

Claire is a self-professed emotional eater. When she is stressed or angry she turns to sweets to get her through the day. Her emotions trigger her eating, and her eating triggers her emotions. A bad day can be followed by a carton of ice cream, which initially makes her happy. Unfortunately, the happiness is short lived and is often followed by waves of guilt, shame, and disappointment. Claire mentally chastises her own behaviour of indulgence, and the sadness sets in. Often this triggers another cycle of eating and the pattern continues. She feels bad—she turns to food—she eats and feels better for a short period of time—she feels worse later on. Claire is a classic emotional eater.

The Calorie Drinker

How much juice do you drink in a day? What do you take in your coffee? How much pop or sugary drinks do you consume? Have you ever stopped to count the calories?

Jim is a thirty-five-year-old type 2 diabetic who came to see me for weight loss. At the time of our first meeting he drank two cans of pop and two glasses of juice per day. Every morning at his coffee break he had an extra large double-double. On weekends he would have a few beers with the guys while watching the game. Jim and I sat down and did the math. Every day he was drinking at least 600 calories in sugar-laden drinks. Jim cut out his juice completely. He switched to one diet pop a day and now uses Splenda and milk in his coffee. On weekends he limits himself to two beers. Jim lost six pounds in the first month in my practice.

Stacey came to her first appointment with her four-year-old daughter, Madeline, in tow. She really wanted to make the appointment and the babysitter was sick. No problem. What was a problem was that Madeline was drinking a juice box. Madeline finished her juice box and asked for another; Stacey provided. Stacey drinks a large caramel frappuccino every morning for breakfast, which means she consumes 1000 calories before she even starts her day. Stacey and I had a long chat. Madeline has not had a juice box since and Stacey treats herself to a small frappuccino on Tuesdays.

The Fast-Food Junkie

Paul is thirty-eight years old and married with two kids. When he was six years old his parents bought him his first Happy Meal and he has never looked back. Paul easily eats out five days a week. He has lunch at a drive-through on a daily basis. His only frame of reference for a hamburger is one that he unwraps. He openly tells me that he dreams about food from McDonald's and Kentucky Fried Chicken. In his own words, they are the food of his childhood—his first great food memories. He has tried to go off fast food cold turkey and has only lasted a week. His usual meal is two double cheeseburgers, a large fries, and a soft drink. He is ashamed and saddened by his inability to give up what he calls an addiction.

The All-or-Nothing Dieter

Melanie has been dieting for decades. She has tried every commercial program available, but the story always ends the same. She starts out a program with perfect intentions and goes to extremes; she will, in her own words, "deny" or "restrict" herself to be "good." This lasts two to three weeks at the most and then she caves—she will not be "denied" any longer. Thereafter begins an eating pattern where she makes up for lost time. It is as though a part of her brain is even more sensitive after the period when she did restrict herself (and science shows it is) and she cannot control her eating. She has only two speeds of dieting—she is at either end of the extremes.

The Portion Distorter

Joanna is twenty-seven years old, and she is seventy-five pounds overweight. She honestly does not know what the problem is. She literally "woke up one morning and had gained fifty pounds." Joanna thinks she eats a healthy diet; she rarely eats out and her food choices are generally healthy. But when Joanna and I do a food audit where she writes down everything she eats it's clear to both of us that she has portion distortion. Although she is eating healthy foods, she's eating too much of them. Joanna's snacks consist of handfuls of almonds. She easily eats six to eight pieces of fruit per day. Volume is Joanna's issue.

The Sitting Duck

Tony is thirty-six years old and hates to exercise. He has a treadmill in his basement that his wife now uses to hang the laundry on. This is not his first piece of home exercise equipment, either. He has been a member of many gyms and has never used their services. At 330 pounds, he does not know where to start. His knees hurt—hell, his whole body hurts! He comes home from his day at the office (where he has a sedentary job) and he is exhausted. All he wants to do is sit on the couch and relax. He would like to be able to walk up a flight of stairs without being out of breath, but he has no idea how to take those first steps toward change.

That was two years ago. Tony now knows that we don't have to like something to do it every day. Tony and I started small, and now he is on his treadmill every night for forty-five minutes while watching the news. He calls it his "me time," where the rest of the world falls away. Tony's progression toward being more active was a slow but definite process. I would argue that because of this slow change and despite life's uncertainties, he will never look back.

So there you have my six Eating Personalities. There must be one or more in each of you, dear reader, so why not get to know yourself a little better? Who knows—you might learn something profound.

I'm not suggesting that who you are is strictly determined by your behaviour. We must, however, acknowledge that human beings are creatures of habit. Who we are is often a reflection of numerous behaviours we engage in on a repeated basis. When it comes to our relationship with food, human behaviour does play a significant role in how we interact with it—our consumption of it, our perceptions of it, and our feelings along the way.

Learning is a complicated set of activities. Some of the best learning, however, happens through error. I would argue that many of my worst mistakes in life were indeed my best lessons. It is therefore essential that we do indeed learn from our mistakes. The point of these Eating Personalities is for us to see a pattern of behaviour, to acknowledge the error, and to make an adjustment in that behaviour.

Most people see flaws as weakness. As you go through these next few chapters, I want you to celebrate your discovery of the imperfections in your behaviour. Remember that once you know where the errors are, you can use them to create a blueprint for the changes you want to make to achieve the ultimate and long-term goal of continued improvement in your relationship with food and your overall health.

3

The Emotional Eater

Do you remember your first birthday cake? I most certainly do. You see, my birthday falls the week after Valentine's Day, and my mother always made me a pink and white valentine cake. If I close my eyes right now, I can taste the vanilla cake with the white icing and the bitterness of the red frosting with the crunch of the cinnamon sweetheart candies that were littered across the top. This is my first sense memory of food.

I am quite sure we all have such a memory. What was the best meal you've ever had? Where did you have your first ice cream cone? What was the best piece of apple pie you've ever tasted? What is your favourite burger place? Who makes the best french fries in town? I ask these questions and immediately you not only have a response, but you have a physiological response. You can taste the icing on your first birthday cake; you savour the sweetness of that first ice cream cone and can describe in detail its taste and its texture and likely even the context in which it was eaten.

There is an emotional component attached to many of our foods in addition to the palatability of them. Culturally, these emotions are embedded in our brains at a very young age. I would argue that the majority of us have some component of emotional eating in our behaviour. Ask the person next to you what their "food weakness" is and you'll get a variety of answers. I think ice cream is the greatest food in the world; for much of my life, if I was having a bad day, ice cream would make it better. I have nursed many disappointments or failures on a couch with a pint of ice cream.

My relationship with ice cream began when I was about four years old. I can remember my first ride to an ice cream parlour in the back seat of my father's Oldsmobile Cutlass Supreme. The seats were as big as a large couch and we did not have to wear seatbelts back in those days. I stood up for almost the entire ride with my face pressed against the window. The promise of ice cream awaited me, and the excitement was more than I could bear. When we arrived at the parlour, my father lifted me up to see all the flavours displayed underneath the glass. There were so many flavours to choose from, but even as a child I was pretty decisive. It was an easy decision: I would have blue licorice. I loved licorice and the ice cream was a bright turquoise colour. How could I go wrong? I can still recall the sweet creamy taste of that ice cream and the hundreds of cones that followed after. Ice cream soon became my "go to" food to make anything better. Why not? When I think about it, as a child, ice cream was associated with happy times, like Sundays in the summer with my family. Any birthday party or celebration, or any time I deserved a treat—all occasions were punctuated with ice cream.

When I was in Grade 6 I had my first boyfriend. His name was Steven, and he liked me for me. (Recall that I was a rather chubby kid in Grade 6.) The fact that I had a boyfriend was a big deal. Steven was really nice to me. He would leave me love notes in my desk at school, and he even invited me to be his date at his brother's wedding. I remember the wedding because it was the day before I got my braces. We had a great time; we danced and drank Shirley Temples, and Steven gave me my first goodnight kiss. The next morning I got my braces put on. My teeth were killing me, and nothing felt good to eat. I was inconsolable. And two days later, Steven broke up with me. My heart was broken and my mouth was in agony. My father picked me up from school and promptly drove me to the ice cream parlour. There was nothing that a blue licorice ice cream could not fix.

This was my emotional eating. Ice cream fixed my breakups and my misgivings. Ice cream never let me down. In university I used ice cream to handle social and academic failures. In residency, if I had a bad day at work, I would sit on the couch with a pint of Häagen-Dazs and let the rest of the world fall away.

Emotional Eating 101

The truth is that there is a physiology behind emotional eating. Remember that our bodies are engineered to maintain a certain level of nutrients for us to survive. Because of this, we have evolved a highly regulated system of circuits that determine how often we feed and on what. In other words, our mealtime habits and patterns are hard-wired into the hypothalamus and the brainstem. The hypothalamus is located just above your brainstem at the base of the brain. It regulates hunger, thirst, sleep, and body temperature and aids in the release of certain sex hormones. The brainstem is in the back of the brain just at the base and is responsible for basic body functions; it keeps your heart beating and your lungs breathing. It is also the control centre of the brain, where all sensory and motor nerve impulses pass through from the spinal cord on their way to the brain.

These two areas of the brain together are the key areas responsible for regulating body weight and are known as the homeostatic system of the brain. They essentially maintain status quo in the body. They perform the functions we really don't think much about and often take for granted (of course, until they stop working properly).[24] This homeostatic system in the brain receives messages from your gut when you are beginning to eat to tell you when you are full. Your brain also receives hunger messages from your stomach and fat tissue to prompt you to eat so that you can adequately maintain a certain level of nutrition for survival.[25]

Ghrelin is the sender of one such message. It is a powerful

hunger hormone that is secreted by the stomach and communicates with the hypothalamus, triggering hunger. As you will see later in this book, ghrelin levels rise within days of starting any caloric restriction as a means of preventing starvation. Your body wants you to eat to stay alive; you are hard-wired to do so.

On the other hand, there are a variety of satiety hormones at work as well (hormones that make you feel full). Leptin is one of the key satiety hormones in the body. It is present both centrally in the hypothalamus and peripherally in fat cells. The bigger your fat cells, the more leptin there is in your system. Leptin acts almost as a messenger system, telling the brain how much energy your body has stored. Think of leptin like the gas gauge on your car: It tells you how much energy is in the tank, and ideally when you should fill up. Unfortunately, it doesn't always work this way. Studies show that the brain has a certain "leptin set point." This means that even though people may have significant body stores of fat, their brain is *used to* a higher level of leptin. When you start to lose weight, your fat cells shrink and your leptin levels fall. Once they fall below that leptin set point, the brain thinks it is starving and signals are sent out to the rest of the system to increase hunger, decrease restraint toward food, and lower certain metabolic responses to activity.[26] You know that little light on the gas gauge of your car that lights up when you have less than an eighth of a tank left? Imagine if it was broken and the light in your car went on when your gas gauge fell below half a tank. Sure, you have more than enough gas to get you where you want to go, but that damn light is on. You've been conditioned to respond to that light. That light must go off, so you stop and fill up. The light goes off and order is restored.

What about people who carry excess fat? If fat cells produce leptin, it would stand to reason that people with excess fat tissue would have higher leptin levels than lean individuals. That is certainly the case. So if leptin is a satiety hormone, one would expect that people who are overweight or obese would have higher levels of satiety or feel more full. Not so. Not only do these people have a higher leptin set point (as explained above), they are also *leptin resistant.*[27] What this means is that these people have high levels of leptin circulating in their bodies, but their brain perceives it as *white noise*—the brain is not getting the higher-leptin message. A great deal of research has been done into leptin resistance and its role in people who are overweight or obese.[28]

Let's go back to our gas-gauge analogy. Imagine driving from Vancouver to Halifax in a car with a broken gas gauge. The gauge on the car says one thing, but the tank always says another. Being a smart problem solver, you would probably work something out. You'd calculate how many litres of gas your tank needed, and then do some pretty savvy math to determine how many kilometres you could drive before filling up the tank. Not bad, right? Now imagine driving from Vancouver to Halifax with a broken gas gauge and severe short-term memory loss. No fancy calculations for you, because you can't remember when you last filled up your car. Finally, imagine the same road trip with a broken gas gauge, short-term memory loss, and the ability to overfill your gas tank by 50 percent. This analogy gives you a bit of an idea about some of the intricacies of the obese brain.

All I have done here is highlight some of the key players in the physiology of hunger and satiety. This still does not explain why certain emotions influence our appetite. Hunger is a basic reflex that, as mentioned, is governed by the homeostatic system in the hypothalamus and brainstem. But in today's world appetite is a learned response.[29] It is governed by the conscious part of our brain, which is in our cortex and receives cues from the world around us—sights, smells, sounds, emotions, memory, and so on.[30] The conscious part of your brain exists in the cortex, including the area of the brain known as the corticolimbic centre. This part of the brain receives messages from the outside world by way of taste, smells, and sensations. Our brain processes these in the corticolimbic centre and stores them in our memory. My birthdays were amazing with fabulous cakes—my cortex saw, smelled, and tasted them and has stored the memories. My brain did not need to rely on primitive homeostatic centres to tell me about my birthday cakes; there were higher functions at work instead.

You see, we live in a world where the majority of us do not need to rely on our primitive nerve network in the brain to fill up the gas tank, so to speak. We have too much food around us, so we no longer need a complex network to tell us when to eat. Because our conscious world has so many food cues—from commercials to advertisements to sights and smells—our conscious brain is constantly reminded about the role food plays in our lives.

Therefore, the corticolimbic centre of the brain now determines much of our current regulation of food intake.[31] This is known as the hedonistic centre of the brain. Studies have shown that in an environment like ours, where food is plentiful, the brain's regulatory centre communicates with its hedonistic centre, and feeding behaviour is now influenced by higher cortical functions. In fact, studies using functional MRI show that this area lights up significantly in response to visual cues to food independent of hunger and satiety. Now our hedonistic part of our brain is telling us when and what to eat, which no longer has anything to do with hunger. We are now at the mercy, so to speak, of our memories, good and bad, in response to food. Our pleasure centre, not our hunger centre, is calling the shots.

Not only is your pleasure centre delegating when and what you eat, but it also gets feedback from the hypothalamus as to what tastes good and what makes you feel good.[32] You store new sensations in your sense memory and create for yourself a wonderful memory bank of what you like and what you don't like. In short, you've got yourself a list of cravings. Add that to a system where your regulation of hunger and satiety is already out of whack and you have a recipe for disaster.

Back to our cross-country road trip. In a world where there is a gas station on every corner, your car no longer operates based on its gas gauge at all. You can fill up anytime you want. Your pit stops are now determined based on when you *feel* like filling up, or based on what your favourite gas station is. Maybe you used Shell in the past and are a fan. Or maybe you have a Petro-Canada card and want the points. You can take your pick. Maybe your car now has a mind of its own and it decides when and where you'll stop. Couple that with a broken gas gauge and a wicked case of short-term memory loss and you have yourself one hell of a ride.

Natasha is a forty-six-year-old woman who has been obese for as long as she can remember. In our first visit together, now three years ago, she told me that her mother put her on her first diet at the age of seven. She describes in vivid detail how she brought a can of tuna to school every day in her lunch, along with a small bag of carrots. She recalls in shame how all of the other children had respectable sandwiches and small packages of cookies wrapped in wax paper. Her lunch was a source of disappointment and humiliation. There, in front of her class, she would use the small can opener included in her lunch bag to open her can of tuna, empty the water, and eat it straight from the can with the fork her mother had packed.

Natasha spent the next two decades on every weight-loss program she could find. Her story is one of constant fluctuation between denying herself certain foods and indulging in others. She constantly uses terms like "good" and "bad" to describe her behaviour around food. And she now associates tuna and vegetables with punishment. Perhaps this stems from her childhood lunches, where these foods were seen as the penance for her disease; Natasha's tuna cans became an equal source of animosity.

But she can describe in equal detail her favourite food—chocolate. Natasha unabashedly loves chocolate. She can talk about chocolate with the same expression on her face as when she is describing an old friend. She can recall moments in her life when her world did not make sense and she would reach for chocolate as an anchor to her sanity.

Natasha's parents divorced when she was eleven. She remembers seeing her father every weekend, and their visit always began with a trip to the candy store. She would be allowed to pick out two chocolate bars and would usually finish them on the car ride home.

When Natasha was in high school she was easily forty pounds heavier than the other girls in her class. Her mother enrolled her in Weight Watchers. She ate a chocolate bar for lunch every day and nothing more. This was her way to keep her weight down and, put in her words, "still be good."

In university, Natasha fluctuated between starvation programs and indulgence. She would spend weekdays eating only cabbage soup, but she would dream about what she was going to eat on the weekend. She would "plan for the cheating," making lists of all the treats wanted. Bad days were punctuated with Kit Kats or Coffee Crisps—she can even recall turning to Baker's Chocolate when absolutely necessary. Chocolate is her drug of choice when the world comes crashing down—and she still has a secret supply in various locations throughout the house.

What is most impressive is that Natasha is not alone. When I first started my obesity clinic we conducted a study that showed 85 percent of obese women presenting to a community-based weight-loss clinic are emotional eaters.[33] This means that they use food in response to emotions—be it sadness, happiness, shame, guilt, anger, or frustration. Natasha is by far more the rule than the exception. In fact, when I look at the physiology of food and the hedonistic approach our brain takes in response to certain tastes, it amazes me that there are not *more* people like Natasha.

There has been a great deal of research in the area of emotional eating and food addiction. Several formal research-based scales have been established to test a person's emotional attachment to food. One such scale, the Yale Food Addiction Scale (YFAS), has made a correlation between certain foods and addictive tendencies.[34] Let's be clear that the YFAS goes beyond just emotional eating, though. This is a tool used to diagnose a more pathological pattern of behaviour than just the simple concept of emotional eating.

I will not elaborate on food addictions here, but rather focus on the broader, more benign concept of emotional eating.

So how do you avoid becoming an emotional eater? Quite simply, you can't. We cannot fix our emotional response to food. Trying to shut off emotional eating is like trying to shut off the part of your brain that causes you to cry during a sad movie—it almost insists that we lose control of our emotions and become detached from them. But this is not a response we necessarily want. I don't want my patients to be emotionally disconnected from the world around them. Furthermore, I would argue that Natasha had years of programming around food and her emotional response to it. To suggest that this can just be reprogrammed is not only naïve, it is unrealistic and cruel. Try this little exercise the next time you find yourself either laughing or crying: STOP. I mean stop right away, as though you were stopping a car. It is difficult, at best.

I cannot change Natasha's feelings about chocolate, but I can help her alter some of her behavioural patterns toward her "drug of choice."

Are You an Emotional Eater?

The first step is to identify yourself as an emotional eater. If you are a woman and you are overweight or obese, there is a pretty good chance that you are an emotional eater. Most North Americans have emotional tendencies toward food to some degree. As a simple test, answer the follow questions:

1. Do you ever use food as a crutch to help you get through things in life?
2. Do you use food as a reward for "good behaviour" or "praise"?
3. Do you indulge in certain foods with the notion of "I need this"?
4. Do you ever eat certain things because you "deserve" them?

5. Do you have certain foods that help you get through difficult times?
6. Do you have a pattern of behaviour of eating on "bad days"?
7. Do you have certain "go to" foods in times of stress, loneliness, or sadness?

It seems all too simple, but a "yes" to any of these questions could mean that you have a component of emotional eating. What this means is that food serves a purpose in your life to address an emotional need. One of the classic examples among women is premenstrual syndrome—many women find they are particularly susceptible to emotional eating at certain times in their menstrual cycle.

The issue with some emotional eaters is that the food has taken over. They cannot control the eating any better than they can control the emotions. But I'm not suggesting this is what they should do. What needs to happen is that we have to minimize the damage.

Most emotional eaters, unless they are true binge eaters, can portion control their period of indulgence. Part of the solution for emotional eaters is to ensure that there is a "plan of action" for how they deal with their emotional eating. The important thing to remember is that everyone is different—there is no pre-set period of time stipulating when a plan needs to be in place. Each person should pick a set period of time that works for him or her. A realistic approach for tackling such behaviour is over a period of a month or so. The key is to go through all the steps of the process and constantly evaluate which areas you need to work on.

Step 1: Make a List of Your Trigger Foods

Emotional eaters have trigger foods, which are foods that trigger overindulgence. For Natasha it is chocolate—she can't be trusted in a room that has any kind of chocolate in it. If there is a box in her house, she will not portion control and will eat the entire box.

So the first step is to make a list of your trigger foods—all the foods you cannot be trusted around when it comes to either portion control or when you are having a period of emotional eating. I make my patients create trigger food lists all the time. This can be done at this very moment. Most emotional eaters can make their list of trigger foods within a few minutes; others need a little bit of time to think things over. If this is the case, take a few days and keep track of a list of foods that you reach for to calm (or buoy) your emotions.

Remember that most trigger foods not only trigger over-indulgence, they also trigger an emotional response after eating them. Emotional eating often has two phases to it, as outlined in Figure 1 below.

The first phase of the emotional eating arch is simply experiencing an emotion. Usually this is a sad or negative emotion that causes

Figure 1 The Emotional Eating Arch

2. An emotion triggers an eating response

1. The Emotion
Sadness
Stress
Guilt
Shame
Loneliness
Etc.

3. The Eating
Ice cream
Cookies
Chocolate
Chips
Etc.

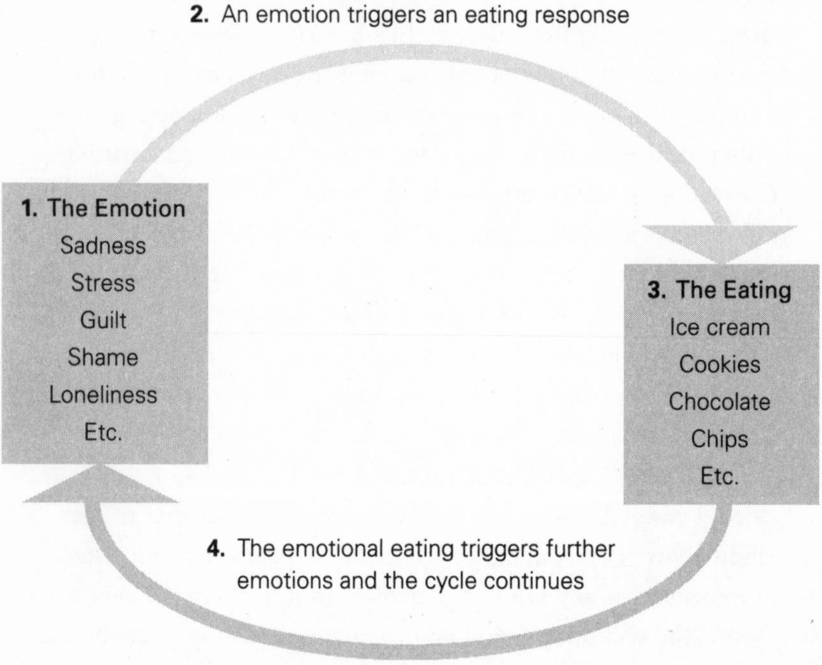

4. The emotional eating triggers further emotions and the cycle continues

you to reach for a trigger food. Natasha has a bad day, and chocolate is her treatment of choice. The next phase to emotional eating is, of course, indulging in the trigger food of choice. Natasha eats two chocolate bars before she even realizes what has happened. Next come the follow-up emotions related to the trigger food. After consuming the food, you feel some kind of negative emotion caused by the indulgence, which often sets off a further set of negative emotions, and the spiral continues.

Natasha feels ashamed about her chocolate indulgence and reaches for another trigger food in the hopes of getting herself out of the slump. This is, of course, followed by further feelings of guilt and shame and the cycle not only continues but also intensifies.

The goal of curtailing emotional eating is not to stop the initial emotion, but to minimize the downward spiral that occurs as a result. As such, the emotional eating no longer spirals out of control and the cycle stops at the second phase. Natasha has a bad day, she eats something in response, but stops the cycle there. How? The answer is forgiveness. When Natasha and others like her stop the cycle at the eating stage and forgive their emotional eating, they minimize the damage and move on. No longer does the emotional eating arch have a continuous component. In this case, the emotional eating cycle would look like Figure 2 on the next page.

The first step to stopping the emotional eating arch is to know what foods trigger the second part of the eating cycle. These, of course, are your trigger foods. For Natasha her list looks like this:

- Chocolate
- Any baked good
- Ice cream
- Granola
- Cashews
- Licorice
- Almonds

Figure 2 Stopping the Emotional Eating Arch

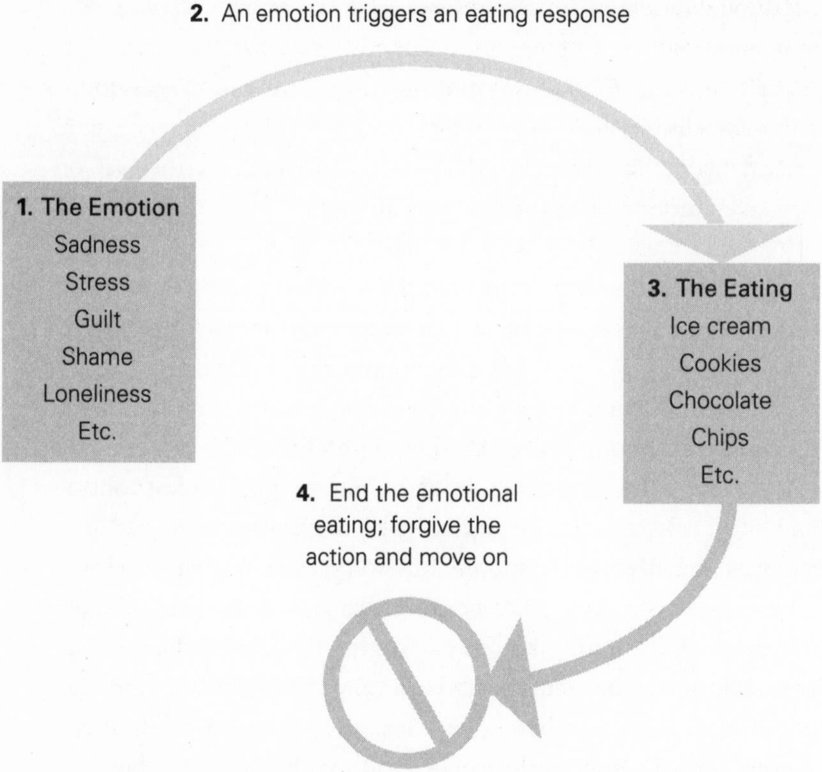

2. An emotion triggers an eating response

1. The Emotion
Sadness
Stress
Guilt
Shame
Loneliness
Etc.

3. The Eating
Ice cream
Cookies
Chocolate
Chips
Etc.

4. End the emotional eating; forgive the action and move on

You'll notice that this list has predominately sweet things on it. You'll also notice that some of those things are not necessarily unhealthy (almonds, granola), but when consumed in large quantities they can really derail healthy eating. Remember that your list may change over time—sometimes the pull of a trigger food wears off, or something new takes its place. So be sure to revisit your trigger food list from time to time; I recommend every couple of months. Update it and evaluate the foods on it.

The real key with trigger foods and emotional eating has to do with their amounts. Remember that when we are talking about breaking the emotional eating cycle we are not talking about abolishing emotional eating entirely. Instead we are talking about *minimizing the damage.* You will not substitute a trigger food for something healthier—that just does not work. If you "need" chocolate to get you through a bad day, there's no way a piece of fruit is going to cut it as a substitute. The key is to remember that one chocolate bar has 250 calories (on average). Have one chocolate bar and move on. Having four chocolate bars is an entirely different story.

Minimizing the damage is part of the second stage of conquering emotional eating: managing the point of entry.

Step 2: Managing the Point of Entry

Here's the deal with trigger foods: If you can't trust yourself in a room with them, never let them in the room. The key with these foods is their point of entry.

Sharon is forty-two years old and is an emotional eater. Her list of trigger foods includes fresh-baked chocolate chip cookies. I ask Sharon how she gets her "fix." She looks at the floor and, almost heartbroken, admits, "I bake them." Sharon does not want to live in a world where she can't have warm chocolate chip cookies, and I don't blame her. But she shouldn't bake the cookies herself. Baking them means she puts herself in a position where she must rely on willpower to stop from eating all of them. Every time she bakes cookies she thinks this time will be different. She tries to make a plan where she will only keep a dozen cookies and put the rest away: She will send them with her son to school; she will take the leftovers to work. Then all her plans go to hell the minute she pulls the first batch from the oven. Sharon's problem is not willpower, it's brain chemistry. Sharon's brain is hard-wired toward this emotional response to warm chocolate chip cookies.

It takes work, but the first step for Sharon is to never bake those cookies again. By doing this, she has stopped the trigger food from entering her house and no longer has to endure the torture that occurs every time she bakes the cookies.

Let's really keep it simple: If a food talks to you, get it out of the house. Don't even go down that aisle in the grocery store. When

Sharon wants a cookie now she has to go out to a bakery and get it. She has made her kitchen much more of a safe place than before. Stop your trigger foods at the door—once you do that, you take "will" out of the equation entirely. You limit the ability of those foods to create further bad emotions; you limit the damage, so to speak, of the emotional eating arch.

Step 3: Eat Treats, Not Treatments

Sharon still loves cookies. They are her treat and she should by no means go without them. Remember when I said she should not live in a world where she can't have fresh-baked cookies? I meant it. But changing the context of how we consume certain foods can, in itself, change our emotional response to them. Sharon loves the ceremony of baking the cookies and how the house smells during the baking. She loves the time she takes out of her life where the world stops and she bakes. She loves the moment when the cookies come out of the oven and sitting at the table eating them. Maybe it takes her back to when she was a kid; maybe it's just the act of doing something for herself. It really does not matter.

The key is that this ritual has become a treatment for Sharon, but she needs to break the cycle. And so for one month we focus on that alone. She puts together a cookie schedule: Twice a week she has treat days, which are planned days where she has a treat. For Sharon her treat is cookies, so twice a week she goes down to her favourite café and buys herself two cookies. She sits at a table with a magazine and a coffee and spends thirty minutes by herself. She has her new ritual in place. She spends time solidifying this ritual, which takes work, but in reality, she is spending much less time on her new ritual than she was on her old one. (Sharon easily baked cookies twice a week.)

If there is a part of you that is an emotional eater, you definitely have your work cut out for you. Remember that each day is a new one; three steps is just the start:

1. Make a list.
2. Cut the foods out at the point of entry.
3. Establish a new ritual around the foods you love so that they are treats and not a treatment.

Finally and most importantly, forgiveness is a vital part of the process. I know that sounds trite, but it is true in any process where change is key—allow yourself to make mistakes and to learn and heal from them. Understand that a big part of emotional eating spiralling out of control depends on how you respond to the mistakes you make. When Sharon and Natasha beat themselves up over their emotional eating, that is when they were doing the most damage. When they forgive their mistakes and learn from them instead, their ability to heal and grow begins. I've seen positive changes happen in the most unlikely of places. We all respond really well to kindness so *never* sell yourself short.

4

The Calorie Drinker

Mathew is what I would call my dream patient. In addition to being a really likeable person, Mathew drinks a lot of his calories. Let me explain.

Mathew is thirty-six years old and the father of three young children. He and I met for the first time more than a year ago when he came to see me for an assessment of his cardiac risk. Every male in Mathew's family had had either a heart attack or a stroke before the age of sixty, and he wanted to know if there was anything he could do to avoid a similar fate. Without getting too far into the details, I did a full history and physical and checked Mathew's blood work, including cholesterol and blood sugars, as well as several other tests to determine his cardiovascular risk profile. When I see a patient it's vital that I get a sense of their eating, drinking, and exercising patterns in addition to their medical and social history. So when I asked Mathew about his eating patterns part of the problem became clear.

The most striking thing about Mathew's pattern of behaviour was the amount of calories he drank in a day. Mathew had one to two glasses of juice per day; in fact, when he added it up, his family of five easily went through 10 litres of juice per week. Mathew drank a can of pop every day with lunch and often another with dinner. At coffee break he would have either a large, fancy coffee with syrups and caramel or a blended coffee in the summer with or without whipped cream. On weekends, Mathew had five or six beers with the guys while watching the game. On Friday nights he and his wife got a sitter and went out to dinner, where they would split a bottle of wine. Mathew and I sat down and did the math:

Mathew's Liquid Calories

Item	Calories per serving	Total calories per week
Orange juice	150 calories per 300 mL glass	1 large 600 mL glass per day = 300 calories × 7 = 2100 calories
Regular pop	180 calories per can	2 cans per day = 360 calories × 7 = 2520 calories
"Fancy coffee," large iced cappuccino	460 calories per 500 mL	1 coffee per day = 460 calories × 7 = 3220 calories
Beer	150 calories per can	6 cans per week = 150 calories × 6 = 900 calories
Wine	120 calories per glass	2–3 glasses per week = 120 × 2 (or 3) = 240–360 calories

When Mathew and I added it all up, he was consuming almost 9000 calories per week in liquids alone. That's equal to drinking more than 2 pounds a week in sugar-laden items.

It's not just that these drinks are bad for Mathew—because they are—the bigger problem is that he is wasting his calories on nutritionally empty foods: Most sugar drinks are nutritionally poor for the amount of calories they "cost." Furthermore, consumption of fructose and high fructose corn syrup (the key ingredient in most sugar-sweetened drinks) has been shown to acutely raise blood pressure in both animals and humans. Long-term consumption of high fructose corn syrup has been linked to the development of high blood pressure, diabetes, and obesity in a variety of studies.[35]

A study published in 2010 in the *Journal of the American Society of Nephrology* looked specifically at this issue.[36] The investigators examined the consumption habits of over 4500 Americans and their overall risk of developing hypertension or high blood pressure. In this cross-sectional analysis, the study showed that more than half of the participants consumed over 75 grams of fructose per day in the form of sweetened drinks. The group with higher fructose consumption was 78 percent more likely to develop hypertension in the coming ten years than the group that consumed much less refined sugar.

The Framingham Heart Study, an observational study of more than 6000 people with an average age of fifty-nine years, provides another example. In one particular aspect of the study, published in *Circulation* in 2007, the authors looked at the relationship between consumption of sugar-sweetened beverages and the development of cardiovascular risk factors.[37] When they controlled for all other variables, the consumption of one or more glasses of pop or juice per day was associated with an 18 percent increased risk in developing hypertension, a 31 percent increased risk of developing obesity, and a 25 percent relative risk of developing borderline diabetes.

Most people would agree that it's no surprise that consuming sugar-sweetened drinks contributes to excess weight gain and the risk factors that go with it. What is shocking is the fact that these sugar-laden substances are by themselves a contributor to hypertension because of their chemical makeup. First, most of these drinks contain large amounts of high fructose corn syrup, which, when broken down by the body into fructose and glucose, produces uric acid. Uric acid has been linked to the development of hypertension and gout.[38] Second, liquid calories have been shown to be less satiating or less filling than solid calories. Several studies have looked at the satiety scales of people after consuming cola, juice, and milk versus eating the same amount of calories and have found that eating fills you up more than drinking. It has been proposed that liquid calories do not trigger the same satiety response in the brain as do solid calories.[39] Finally, liquid calories are pretty expensive, so to speak. As an exercise, the table below highlights some caloric equivalents for some of the most common, everyday drinks.

Liquid Calories vs. Solid Calories[40]

Drink	Calories consumed	Healthier food option for the same amount of calories	Unhealthier food option for the same amount of calories
Grande mocha with whipped cream	330	Turkey sandwich	Bean burrito
Grande caramel frappuccino with whipped cream	390	Chicken breast with salad and 1/2 cup of sweet potatoes	Sausage McMuffin
Venti caramel macchiato	300	6 ounces of grilled salmon, salad, and a piece of bread	8 chicken nuggets
Beer (1 can)	150	1 apple and 1 ounce of cheese	15 M&Ms
Cola (1 can)	180	1/2 piece of whole-wheat pita with 2 tbsp of hummus	Small crunchy taco
Hot chocolate with whipped cream (medium)	360	Cobb salad, no dressing, no bacon	Burger King small cheeseburger
Gin and tonic	200	Half a cantaloupe with cottage cheese	Half a cup of Häagen-Dazs ice cream
Juice	150	1 banana, 1 orange	2 Oreo cookies

I know Mathew may seem like an extreme, but I suspect he is more the rule than the exception. The big question facing Mathew and those like him is, "How do I give it up?" The answer is *slowly,* and below I'll show you how Mathew scaled back on his liquid calories.

First off, I'm not suggesting that Mathew immediately put down the pop and the juice and the fancy coffees and drink water for the rest of his life. I do, however, think there is a way for him to slowly transition to a way of eating (and more importantly, drinking) that is much better for him and that does not waste so many of his calories on nutrient-poor, high-calorie, high-sugar beverages.

The sections below outline two ways to redecorate your calorie drinking. Remember that each of the steps included in each method can be done over a few weeks to a month. I suggest that you make one change once a month and build upon each one. As with everything, try one method at a time and see how it works for you. You may find that you need to alternate between the two methods before you find one that works.

Quick Changes

1. **Cut out all juice.** Manufacturers make you think it's healthy for you, all full of pulp, vitamins, and natural ingredients, but when you juice a fruit you take away all of the fibre, leaving only sugar and some vitamins. In fact, the juice contained in fruits is nature's way of getting you to eat the fibre in the first place! Remember, juice is just pop with a multivitamin.
2. **If you must drink pop, switch to diet pop.** Make no mistake—diet pop has its own controversies, and water is always best, but to tell someone who drinks three cans of pop a day to switch to water is unrealistic. Perhaps a better "weaning process" is to move from regular pop to diet pop, and then after a while move to water.
3. **Fancy coffees?** Choose lower-calorie alternatives. Get rid of the whipped cream, switch to low-fat milk, and use sugar-free sweeteners. Find a way to lower the calories in the drinks you like by cutting the quantity and trimming the fat and sugar.

4. **Size does matter, so downsize your sugary drinks.** If you are drinking a large, switch to a medium for a few weeks, and then ultimately to a small. You'll eliminate anywhere from 200 to 1000 calories just by downsizing, depending on the drink.
5. **What about alcohol?** Alcohol is full of empty calories. If you have to have a drink before dinner, try and stick with a lower-calorie alternative. Mixed drinks are the worst offenders; below is a chart of common alcoholic mixed drinks and their caloric content, so pick a lower-calorie alternative. Alternatively, you can use a sugar-free or lower-calorie mixer. For example, vodka with club soda and lemon juice would contain far fewer calories than vodka and orange juice. Finally, as a rule, try to restrict your alcohol consumption to no more than one to two drinks per week.

Drink	**Calories per serving**
Piña colada	645
Margarita	300–450
Martini	150
Fancy cocktail (mojito, cosmopolitan, bellini, etc.)	200–450
Caesar or Bloody Mary	160
Gin and tonic	120
1 ounce alcohol with a regular mixer (rum and Coke, rye and Coke, vodka and cranberry juice, etc.)	150–200
Beer	200
Glass of wine or champagne	120
1 ounce of 80-proof alcohol on the rocks (e.g., scotch, bourbon, vodka)	80
1 ounce alcohol with diet mixer (e.g., rum and Diet Coke)	80

Slow Changes

1. **Make a list of all the beverages you drink in a day.** You can see that when Mathew and I did the math it was eye-opening, so take a moment and calculate what you drink in a day. Multiply your calories by seven days and you have the amount of calories you drink in a week. You also have a place to start making changes.
2. **Establish a daily caloric budget for drinking your calories.** As a starting point, cut what you are drinking daily in half. If we take an example from Mathew, here's how we make a liquid budget:

Mathew's Liquid-Calorie Budget

Item	OLD Mathew	NEW Mathew	Calories saved
Orange juice	600 mL a day (300 calories)	300 mL per day (150 calories)	150 cal/day 1050 cal/week
Regular pop	2 cans per day (360 calories)	Diet pop (0–7 calories)	360 cal/day 2520 cal/week
"Fancy coffee", large iced cappuccino	500 mL a day (460 calories)	Tall iced cappuccino with milk (200 calories)	260 cal/day 1820 cal/week
Beer	6 cans on Sunday (900 calories)	4 cans on Sunday (600 calories)	300 cal/week
Wine	2–3 glasses (120 calories per glass)	2–3 glasses (120 calories per glass)	0

From Mathew's perspective, he's cut out 5690 calories in a week, mostly by switching to diet pop and downsizing his drinks. Remember that you don't have to make these changes all at once. These changes can be slower and more systematic. I often tell patients to do one change a month.

The key with these changes is to continue. Once you've cut your budget in half, wait a couple of months to let the changes stick. Then you can re-evaluate your budget again and see where you can cut things further.

3. **Establish some "deal breakers" and make a plan for how to enjoy them responsibly.** Once you've modified your calorie-drinking budget you'll need to be clear about your deal breakers. These are the drinks that you just do not want to live without, and I don't think you should. But I want you to enjoy them healthfully. Perhaps it is your large morning latte with vanilla syrup—switch to a smaller size and go for a sugar-free option.

Mathew's deal breaker is the wine he shares with his wife on weekends. For me, it's my soy latte. With deal breakers, you need to establish if you can modify them at all or if they stand as they are. Mathew likes the wine he has with his wife, but he is sticking with two glasses. As for me, I used to drink two to three soy lattes daily. I don't want to live without my coffee, but I have changed my soy latte to a small and it happens with brunch on Sundays. I still drink three coffees daily, but now they are plain coffees with just a splash of soy milk; a small way to redecorate.

4. **Continue to modify your drinking habits on a regular basis.** Pick a time frame that you can work with and modify, modify, modify. As for Mathew? After about six months he gave up fancy coffees and switched to plain coffee with milk. A few months later he completely cut out juice. The point is that Mathew's changes sparked a positive cycle in his life and his approach to calorie drinking.

Calorie drinking on the surface seems like an obvious behavioural change that can be made easily. But like any habit, it can be hard to break. Be patient with your habits and always stop for a minute and see where you are on your path to change. Getting derailed can happen—you may find yourself a few months into new habits, and out of nowhere you are drinking your calories again. Be aware of your patterns of behaviour and where there is room for change. Sure, it won't be easy, but I suspect you are up for the task.

5

The Fast-Food Junkie

When you read about Jake, many of you will think I am lying. In fact, I must preface this chapter by saying that Jake is very real. Of course I have changed some of the details of all the patients in this book to preserve their privacy, but apart from the name and a few identifying features, Jake really does exist. In fact, I would argue that people like Jake are more common than we think.

Jake is thirty-eight years old. He is a lawyer, he lives alone, and he eats out every day of his life. On weekdays he has a Tim Hortons breakfast sandwich for breakfast along with a large latte. For lunch he goes to the food court attached to his office building for Chinese food, a hamburger, or soup and a sandwich. For dinner he orders pizza or visits a drive-through. On weekends he usually eats out with friends and spends Sunday nights at a pub with friends watching a game.

Jake eats almost every meal outside of his home. He is a fast-food junkie. Jake tells me that it began innocently enough. He started working at his law firm and found no time to make his meals, and he had never been a fan of cooking in the first place. As a kid, his parents always had family dinners. When he went away to university, the family dinners stopped and pizza became his food group—fast food was part of his university culture. When he began articling at his first firm, many nights were spent working at the office and the firm would order in.

His environment slowly began to conform to the convenience of fast food, which became the norm. When Jake got his first job at a law firm as an associate he thought some of the patterns he had developed over the years might change. But in retrospect, he'd been eating fast food at least four or five days a week for over a decade. Now at thirty-eight, he sees the food as a convenience and the only thing he knows.

Change is a challenge on any level. Hearing Jake's story may seem surreal to those of us who rarely eat out, let alone at a fast-food restaurant. But in reality Jake is just "one of the guys." According to Eric Schlosser's book, *Fast Food Nation*, 25 percent of Americans eat fast food daily.[41] As Canadians, we often like to think we are different than our neighbours to the south, but we are not. In 2004, the Canadian Community Health Survey asked 35,000 people what they had eaten in the previous 24 hours: More than 25 percent reported eating or drinking something from a fast-food restaurant. Among teenagers ages 14–18, the number was as high as 35 percent. More than 40 percent of the people surveyed opted for a pizza, hamburger, or hot dog, and 25 percent of them washed things down with a sugar-sweetened drink.[42]

The latest available data on fast-food consumption and spending comes from the 2007 World Population Data Sheet. The numbers, based on 2004 data, show that Canada ranks number three in the world for fast-food spending, shelling out $12.7 billion per year on fast food. In 2004, Canadians spent $387 per capita on fast food, making us second only to the Americans in per capita spending (who spend $492 per capita).[43] Further data from Canada's Office of Consumer Affairs shows that only 25 percent of Canadians eat a meal that is cooked for them at home every night. The remaining 75 percent rely on restaurants, fast food, or pre-prepared or prepackaged food.[44]

Jake may be an extreme example, but the rest of the country is not far behind. Jake and I have a chat. This, of course, is an understatement—Jake and I spend several visits, hours in fact, looking at the type of fast foods he eats and where and how to modify this behaviour.

As you have likely realized by now, the plan is not to have Jake begin cooking all of his meals at home and abandoning eating out forever. In fact, Jake has tried this. He's tried several diets where he had to cook and prepare his own meals—he lasted about a week on each. He turned to a meal delivery service, which, in theory, seemed like a great idea; he didn't have to cook and he was eating out anyway, so why not have someone else prepare a healthier version of his "happy meal"? The problem was Jake got bored with the food choices and found that, quite frankly, his palate missed the taste of his unhealthier staples. In short, he missed the Chinese food and the burgers and fries. The grilled chicken and stir-fries he was getting from the healthier meal delivery service just weren't satisfying a brain that had spent a good part of his life adapting to a certain amount of sugar, fat, and salt.

Here's how I tackle the fast-food junkie: Eliminate the excess and modify the must-haves. Essentially, what you are going to do is track your fast-food choices and systematically eliminate them.

Eliminate the Excess

Like Jake, anyone who has spent a good part of his or her life eating restaurant food or fast food can't just give it up overnight. Studies show that our brains adapt very quickly to the palatability or taste of just the right amount of sugar, fat, and salt, and the fast-food industry has spent decades researching this very idea. If we are going to make an impact on our fast-food practices we first need to see what we are up against in our own homes.

Step 1: Make a Food Diary

As with any of my Eating Personalities, the fast-food junkie needs to identify the problem in further detail. The best way to track your eating is to keep a food diary. A food diary is not a way to police your food choices, but rather a blueprint for change. Let's take it step by step, with Jake as our example. I sent Jake home with instructions to keep a food diary for at least one week. Jake's food diary looked like the one on the next page.

Step 2: Highlight the Fast-Food Choices

With the fast-food junkie, we highlight the places where fast food is being consumed. Jake's food diary looks like the one on page 56 after we highlight all the meals he is eating at fast-food restaurants.

Unfortunately, with Jake this is an easy task (as I mentioned before, Jake is an extreme case). Jake's diary is not typical, but as you can see we've only highlighted his fast-food-menu items, even though most of the non-highlighted items are still meals eaten out. The key with Jake is to take it one step at a time.

If you are someone who does not eat fast food, but who does eat restaurant food quite frequently, you may want to try this exercise but highlight the meals that you have eaten in a restaurant instead. This will allow you to look at your "ordering patterns" when you eat out. Once you see what you tend to order at a restaurant you can plan strategies to change your ordering practices.

Step 1: Jake's Food Diary

	Sunday	Monday	Tuesday	Wednesday	Thursday	Friday	Saturday
Breakfast	Skipped	Tim Hortons breakfast sandwich Large latte	Tim Hortons breakfast sandwich Large latte	Tim Hortons breakfast sandwich Large latte	Tim Hortons breakfast sandwich Large latte	Tim Hortons breakfast sandwich Large latte	French toast 2 sausages
Lunch		Chicken Caesar salad	McDonald's cheeseburger meal	Wendy's oriental chicken salad	Pizza sub Soup	Chinese meal for one	Italian panini sandwich Soup
Dinner	Spaghetti and meatballs Salad Breadsticks	Steak Baked potato Caesar salad 2 glasses of wine	Pizza	Pizza	Chinese meal for one	Sushi	Burger Fries 2 beers
Snack		M&M's	Apple	Kit Kat	Chips		

Step 2: Jake's Diary—Fast Food Highlighted

	Sunday	Monday	Tuesday	Wednesday	Thursday	Friday	Saturday
Breakfast	Skipped	Tim Hortons breakfast sandwich Large latte	Tim Hortons breakfast sandwich Large latte	Tim Hortons breakfast sandwich Large latte	Tim Hortons breakfast sandwich Large latte	Tim Hortons breakfast sandwich Large latte	French toast 2 sausages
Lunch		Chicken Caesar salad	McDonald's cheeseburger meal	Wendy's oriental chicken salad	Pizza sub Soup	Chinese meal for one	Italian panini sandwich Soup
Dinner	Spaghetti and meatballs Salad Breadsticks	Steak Baked potato Caesar salad 2 glasses of wine	Pizza	Pizza	Chinese meal for one	Sushi	Burger Fries 2 beers
Snack		M&M's	Apple	Kit Kat	Chips		

Step 3: Modify All Meals Outside the Fast-Food Norm

The next step is to modify all meals that are outside what I would call the *fast-food norm*. For example, breakfast is not usually a fast-food norm. When we think of fast food, for most of us it is lunches at a food court, ordering takeout for dinner, or going to a drive-through window after work. Breakfast does not usually factor into this equation. However, if you are a fast-food junkie who only eats breakfast out, you are in luck—breakfast is probably the best and easiest meal to modify. The key factor with modifying breakfasts is that it really is all about convenience. Find a morning meal that takes less than three minutes to prepare and can, if necessary, be eaten on the run.

Jake and I come up with four fast and easy alternatives for his usual breakfast sandwich:

1. Instant oatmeal
2. Whole-wheat toast with peanut butter and a banana, or a whole-wheat bagel with tomato and cheese
3. A high-fibre, low-sugar cereal with milk and a banana
4. A protein bar

Jake prefers instant oatmeal and he keeps a box at work where he just has to add hot water and can eat it at his desk. The whole-wheat toast or bagel sandwich is often a grab-and-go alternative and eaten en route to work. The cereal is a bit more labour intensive, since Jake usually has to sit down to eat it, but the protein bar works perfectly for the days when he just can't find those extra few minutes in the morning. In fact, he keeps an extra stash of protein bars at work in case of emergency. (I recommend a protein bar with no more than 300 calories and at least 18 to 20 grams of protein.) After two months, Jake's food diary now shows signs of serious improvement.

Make no mistake, this is a slow process. But remember that Jake (like many of you reading this) has tried the quick way and it has

Step 3: Jake's Improved Food Diary

	Sunday	Monday	Tuesday	Wednesday	Thursday	Friday	Saturday
Breakfast	2 pieces of toast with peanut butter Latte	Oatmeal Banana Small non-fat latte	Oatmeal Banana Small non-fat latte	Oatmeal Banana Small non-fat latte	Oatmeal Banana Small non-fat latte	Oatmeal Banana Small non-fat latte	2 pieces of toast with peanut butter Latte
Lunch		Turkey sandwich	McDonald's cheeseburger meal	Wendy's oriental chicken salad	Pizza sub Soup	Chinese meal for one	Turkey sandwich
Dinner	Spaghetti and meatballs Salad Breadsticks	Sushi	Pizza	Pizza	Sushi	Sushi	Burger Fries 2 beers
Snack	Protein bar	Orange	Apple	Apple	Protein bar	Granola bar Yogurt	2 tangerines

not worked. Weight loss is not like pulling off a bandage: You don't rip it quickly and hope for the best. It is like any change—a labour-intensive and patient process. Lifestyle changes are like building a relationship: slow, arduous, and constantly needing attention. As I did with Jake, I recommend making these changes over a period of months. Jake's modification of his breakfasts took a month, and the next month we tackled his lunches.

Modify the Must-Haves

The problem with lunches is that they are often eaten out, so I'm a big fan of packing a lunch. In fact, I would argue that most of the excess calories we accumulate come from mindless choices made while eating out at lunch. This is where the real hazards for the fast-food junkie emerge. Lunches are often plagued by a "quick fix" mentality. For many of us, there is a sense that you have to grab something quickly and get back to work, and this is where the danger truly lies. When we have this quick fix mentality, we are less likely to plan ahead and less likely to make healthier choices. In other words, we are more vulnerable to the elements, to the pull of unhealthy food cues that exist all around us. This is where the pull of fast food becomes greatest—it is quick, easy, inexpensive, and it tastes good.

When we are talking about modifying lunches, Jake and I are faced with one of three options.

Option 1: Pack a Lunch

Jake and I come up with four different "go to" lunches he can prepare quickly at home and take to work. I know what you're thinking: You don't have time to buy the groceries and make your own lunch. I get it, but these four lunches take thirty minutes of shopping once a week and maybe five minutes to make. If this is too much time to invest then, sure, Option 1 is not for you, but give it a try. It's only an extra hour a week of work to really change your life. I bet you can find the time.

Four Lunch Options

1. **The traditional bag lunch.** This is the lunch your mom made you every morning for school. It includes the old favourites, like a peanut butter, turkey, tuna, or cheese sandwich. Lunches don't have to be elaborate. They really can look like the brown bag lunch your mom made you in grade school: a sandwich, a couple of pieces of fruit, a bag of carrots, and you are set. I understand that many people don't have time to shop for groceries, but it doesn't take a lot of extra time and it's well worth it. Buying sandwich supplies, fruit, and some vegetables takes about thirty minutes once a week. If you don't have time for this, then we really need to talk.
2. **The leftover.** This is last night's dinner in a container with a piece of fruit. It can be reheated (every office has a microwave) and you are good to go.
3. **The grab bag.** This is a grab bag consisting of what's in the pantry. A protein bar, a piece of fruit, some cheese and crackers, and some vegetables. The grab bag is what's at home and what's easy, and it involves no cooking. It is literally five food groups thrown in a bag and hoping for the best. Take a bag and put fruit, yogurt, cheese, crackers, and some carrots in and you have an ideal grab bag.
4. **The prepack.** This is a prepackaged meal that is usually frozen. I'm not a huge fan of these options, since they are often high in salt and preservatives, but when compared to fast food they are definitely the lesser evil. This would involve lower-calorie frozen meals or low-sodium canned or instant soups. Remember to add a piece of fruit, a yogurt, and some baby carrots and you've got yourself a pretty decent lunch.

Jake still wants to eat lunch out a few days a week. I don't expect him to pack a lunch every day, at least not right away. This is an ideal long-term goal, but not one I expect him to make right away. This point brings us to Jake's other option.

Option 2: The Lesser Evil

I spoke above about the "lesser evil," which is a second option for the fast-food junkie's lunch. A lesser evil is the fast-food junkie's way of transitioning toward healthier eating; it may not be the "perfect choice," but it is certainly a healthier one than the initial fast-food option. The following table gives you a stepwise process

Jake's Lunch Options

Old option	Healthier option	Even healthier option	Calories saved
Two slices of pepperoni pizza (600 calories)	Lean Cuisine personal deluxe pizza (340 calories)	6-inch grilled turkey club sandwich on whole wheat (320 calories)	260 280
Chinese meal for one (950 calories)	Wonton soup—hold the wontons (400 calories)	Stir-fry vegetables, light on the oil, with brown rice (350 calories)	550 600
Burger and large fries (900 calories)	Burger and salad (600 calories)	Veggie burger and salad (440 calories)	300 460
12-inch pizza sub (900 calories)	6-inch pizza sub (450 calories)	6-inch turkey or ham sub with a lot of veggies (280 calories)	450 620
Fried chicken sandwich (560 calories)	Grilled chicken sandwich (370 calories)	Grilled chicken salad, dressing on the side (310 calories)	190 250
Tempura, 6 pieces Sushi, 8 pieces (1080 calories)	Sushi, 6 pieces California roll, 6 pieces Tuna roll (480 calories)	Sashimi (9 pieces, salmon) and a salad (400 calories)	600 680

to choosing the lesser evil. You will see that in the "Healthier Option" column the items are likely still eaten at the same fast-food restaurant where the old option was picked up. In the "Even Healthier Option" column you are modifying things even further. Some people prefer to just make the "big switch"; others want a stepwise progression. I leave it to you to decide how to remodel your behaviour—there is no right answer.

Option 3: Get Religion

When I say "get religion," I am referring to making a radical change: One day you are a fast-food junkie, and the next morning you wake up a new person who never touches it again. This, of course, would be ideal—Jake gives up fast food entirely and starts taking healthy, nutritious lunches. For those of you who need a "ground shaker" this might be the option you choose.

A radical change is an option, but it is neither common nor necessary in the long run. At best 20 percent of the people I see are able to make a significant, sudden, and permanent change when it comes to fast food. If you are someone who is sick of the old fast-food cycle and want to give it up entirely, you might be the perfect person to jump right in and, yes, get religion. If it does not work for you, then you have the above two options to fall back on. What is really interesting about this final option is that most people who've been doing the above two options repeatedly eventually do move toward this final option.

So Jake, our fast-food junkie, now has three options to change his pattern of behaviour in pursuit of healthier options. He can take lunches, try healthier fast-food alternatives when he does eat out, or he can drastically get religion and make a huge change in his patterns. What's most important to remember about these options is that you can pick and choose among all three on a daily or even weekly basis.

As the months pass, Jake's lunches are more in keeping with a combination of the first two options outlined above. As for Jake's dinners, the plan of attack remains similar to the options he faced regarding his lunches.

The Fast-Food Dinner Makeover

When it comes to making over a fast-food dinner, the key is to highlight what I call the deal breakers. Three years ago I became involved in Diane's care. Diane is a busy mom of four children who has struggled with her weight for many years, but noticed that after she had her kids things really got out of control. In addition to being a full-time mom, Diane also works full-time at a bank. At our first visit she tells me how, between work and the kids and all the responsibilities, she and her husband are just trying to stay alive. She makes lunches for herself and her kids, but dinnertime is an issue. Most days she gets home at 6 P.M. and the last thing she wants to do is cook dinner. Three nights a week the kids have lessons or hockey practice, and she usually finds that the drive-through is the easiest solution. Diane needs to make over her dinners.

Pack Dinner

This is just like packing a lunch. Diane's family is on the move. Her kids take lunch to school but on the nights that they are at lessons somehow a drive-through factors into the equation. I suggest to her that she could also pack dinner for the kids. It is extra work, perhaps, but no more than making dinner at home. She does not have to pack dinner every night that the kids have lessons. We reach an agreement that once a week she'll pack dinner, once a week she will go for a healthier fast-food option like turkey subs on whole-wheat bread, and once a week she and the kids can have a burger, but instead of fries they could go for some cut-up veggies and fruit.

By making small changes like this, what you're doing is putting you back in control of a situation that makes you feel powerless. Life is fast paced, so making a small change instead of going to extremes allows for some wiggle room when things get a little hectic. If you are like Diane, think about what modifications you could make to the fast-food, hockey-mom roller coaster you are currently on.

1. Can you pack dinner once a week?
2. Can you take your kids to a healthier fast-food restaurant?
3. How can you minimize the unhealthier fast-food options that are part of the driving and errands and lessons your family has scheduled?

Make a list of some options and put them into action. Allow for some error and try to be flexible—change does not happen overnight. You may not get it right the first time around, but don't give up. In the long run, both your family and you will benefit.

Pizza Night

Kaycee and her family are a pizza family. At least twice a week they order pizza. Kaycee tells me it is an easy and inexpensive alternative to cooking. Her family is on a fixed income, and she has found that many of the healthy alternatives in the grocery store are more expensive and a bit cost prohibitive. The other issue with pizza night is that Kaycee often orders enough for leftovers for the next day or so. When we really work it out, Kaycee's family is eating pizza easily four days a week. When I ask Kaycee what a typical pizza night involves, she tells me quietly and almost ashamedly that she orders three pizzas, cheesy bread, and chicken wings.

I don't think Kaycee is the exception. Takeout is a common occurrence in North America. Many families find it to be a low-cost and convenient alternative to eating out. Data from my patients show that families order in on average once a week. The majority of these takeout meals are pizza or Chinese food.

Choice and *volume* are key when it comes to takeout food. I'm not asking you to stop eating takeout entirely, but there is a lesson in Kaycee's example. Pizza night does not have to turn into a buffet experience—pizza night can be just pizza, without the cheesy bread, chicken wings, and whatever else might be on the takeout menu. Make sure it is no more than once a week, and order just enough for one family dinner—no leftovers.

In Kaycee's case, she has three young boys. Each boy is allocated two pieces of pizza, and we allocate two pieces for her and three for her husband. We do the math and realize we need twelve slices of pizza, so Kaycee now orders an extra-large pizza for her family. We cut out the cheesy bread and replace it with a salad; the chicken wings are gone entirely. Now pizza night at Kaycee's house is relatively benign compared to its previous state. It's not perfect, but we don't want perfection—we want something that Kaycee and her family can realistically live with that is part of the solution and not part of the problem.

When it comes to takeout try the following:

Step 1: Find the Deal Breaker and Minimize the Damage

Look at what you currently order and isolate the item that you must have. We all have favourites (my husband, Jason, thinks ginger beef is proof of a higher power), but look at what you can cut out or minimize. Find the deal breaker. For my husband it's the ginger beef, and for Kaycee it's the pizza. These are the items that you will not cut out, but the rest can be reworked. Jason orders ginger beef but has steamed vegetables with it instead of honey garlic chicken balls; Kaycee now has pizza and a salad.

Step 2: Size Matters

Particularly with takeout, the larger-size items are often less expensive; the difference between a small pizza and an extra-large one is marginal. That being said, don't think of the money you are saving—think of your and your family's health, which you are investing in by ordering a smaller quantity. Kaycee actually cut her weekly pizza bill in half.

Step 3: Try a Healthy Alternative

This is definitely a more advanced step, but one that you might want to try. For example, Kaycee and her family now order pizza one day a week, and on another night they have homemade-pizza night. She buys whole-wheat pita bread and uses lots of veggies, low-fat cheese, and leftover toppings from the fridge. The fun part is that the kids get to make their own pizza and the event becomes a family affair. Look at what you are eating for takeout and try to modify things as a family. You will find that it is more seamless than you imagined and you really are ordering health off the menu.

Overall, a fast-food junkie is often seen as the easiest Eating Personality to change. Most people perceive that those who eat out all the time can just stop. Understand that behaviours are a part of our general makeup—they are an expression of who we are. Fast-food junkies reflect the society we live in. Restaurants are not going away, and the fast-food culture is here to stay. That being said, you do not have to settle for a substandard nutritional profile just because of time constraints. Like any behaviour change, make some choices, start somewhere, and keep moving forward. There are endless solutions and alternatives to choose from. Engage in the ones that make sense to you, and feel free to problem solve through a few of your own.

6

The All-or-Nothing Dieter

Caroline is a relatively new patient to me. Her problem is one that I see every day and that has essentially fuelled the dieting industry over the decades: Caroline is an all-or-nothing dieter.

She is thirty-eight years old and by her own admission she has been dieting for decades. She started her first diet when she was eight years old and her mother took her to Weight Watchers; she was the youngest person in the group. In fact, she tells me that her mother had to get a special letter from their pediatrician to enroll Caroline in the program. Sound familiar?

Caroline spent the next decade on one diet or another. The pattern was always the same: She would be very strict in following a diet that was inevitably a restrictive program for a period of time and then she would, in her own words, "cheat." She would fall off track and indulge. As a teenager she would be scolded for cheating and it became a judgment call in her home whether she was being "good" or "bad" on her diet. Caroline grew up with a sense of morality attached to whether or not she was following her diet of the day. This way of thinking has persisted many years later.

Caroline continued to diet throughout her twenties and thirties and has been back to Weight Watchers more times than she can count. She has tried every commercial diet available and has bought every book there is and tried to follow the programs outlined in each of them. Caroline's dieting pattern remains the same but has become more extreme as she has gotten older.

Caroline always starts a diet program with vigour. She signs up for the given diet or buys the latest diet book and reads the book as though it were gospel. In her mind, "This is the day it will all come together." She tells herself over and over that "This time will be different." This time she will stick to the program and lose the weight.

But here's the thing. Caroline is really good at following a program, but only for a period of time. Each time she tries a new program she lasts about three to six months at the most. She usually loses between twenty-five and forty-five pounds in this period of time. Once, on a serious starvation program that was very strict, she lost fifty-eight pounds in almost five months. But like any restrictive program she cannot maintain it for a long period of time, and as such the results she achieves are temporary. As Caroline explains, she inevitably falls off track. Something happens in her life to derail her, and she loses focus. Sometimes it's a crisis that takes her off track.

When Caroline was thirty-two she began Jenny Craig. She bought the meals religiously and met with her counsellor weekly. Inside of five months, Caroline had lost forty-five pounds. She felt amazing. She was going to the gym four days a week and was really happy with the program. She liked the food that Jenny Craig had and could see herself keeping this weight off. "This time," she told herself, "would indeed be different." And then her husband lost his job and finances became a problem. As the only breadwinner in the family for a period of time, Jenny Craig became a luxury the family could not afford. She tried buying prepackaged meals at the grocery store from Lean Cuisine or Weight Watchers and creating a makeshift program of her own, but between working full-time and the stress in her home life, the program soon gave way. It took Caroline eighteen months to gain the weight back. She stopped going to the gym and stopped exercising entirely.

Fortunately Caroline's husband found a new job soon after he was let go. But she tells me that by that time, she had lost "that feeling" and had let everything go. Her motivation had disappeared and it was as though she was waiting for a moment when her motivation would return. She would spend days trying to start over and never be able to maintain the momentum that she'd once had. Eventually she just stopped trying altogether. "It was just so hard to get back on track," she says. "I was waiting for a light to go on and it never did."

Caroline continued her dieting seesaw with a variety of commercial, over-the-counter, book-based programs. She would buy the book, read the program, and try it for two to three weeks. Then life happened and the book went back on the shelf.

A few years ago Caroline's sister got engaged and she was determined to lose weight for the wedding. She joined an extreme high-intensity program that consisted of eating only 800 calories a day and injections of vitamins three days a week. She had to weigh in three days a week, and if her weight went up her calories were dropped further to 600 a day. Caroline spent five months on this program. She tells me that at the time she was highly motivated: "I was unstoppable. I found the whole process really easy. I wasn't really hungry and I knew I had a goal." After five months she was down fifty-eight pounds. At her sister's wedding she was bombarded with compliments about how good she looked. She felt amazing. She had accomplished her goal. She had stuck to the program and had lost the weight.

The following week she stopped going to the program. To this day she cannot recall why she stopped going to appointments and following the program. She tells me in recalling that time, "it was just like the switch went off and I lost my motivation. I felt great and even though I think there was a part of me that knew that I had to continue with some program, I just didn't have it in me to continue. I had worked so hard and I was tired. I missed all the food I couldn't have and didn't have for all that time. And so I just stopped following the program." It took Caroline less than a year to gain the weight back. Now, one year later, she sits in my office.

I know that there is a part of Caroline that thinks that I am just her next great diet. Caroline is not only a serial dieter, but she is also a classic example of the all-or-nothing dieter. When she is not on a diet program she is almost out of control. With Caroline there is no in-between—she is either eating prepackaged foods that are portioned out and calorie controlled or she is eating whatever she wants. If I can play dime-store psychologist for a moment, Caroline grew up with a polarity toward dieting and food that has persisted into her adulthood. She was either behaving on her diet or cheating on it: She was "on" or "off," foods were "good" or "bad," and now as an adult she is "all" or "nothing."

What do you do if you are a person like Caroline? As with any of my Eating Personalities, first you have to find out if you are one of them. So, are you an all-or-nothing dieter?

An all-or-nothing dieter is someone who is more than just a serial dieter. An all-or-nothing dieter lives in extremes of behaviour—patterns that cannot fit into their current lifestyle and are, even under the best intentions, doomed to fail. An all-or-nothing dieter has typically been on many programs and is very diet savvy. They have tried a variety of weight-loss techniques from book-based programs to various weight-loss strategies. They have also usually tried a variety of over-the-counter medications for weight loss.

The all-or-nothing dieters have been the fuel behind the commercial weight-loss industry for decades. They have repeatedly beaten themselves up over not being able to adhere to the strict codes of conduct that have been outlined for them. All-or-nothing dieters see food as either good or bad. They have polarized the entire process of being on a weight-loss program; a diet has become that which they fear because it represents yet another future failure.

I would argue that all-or-nothing dieters are the hardest people to treat. It's one thing to change a person's behaviour—we do this all the time in our everyday lives, because we have rules and codes of conduct that affect how people act—but it is another matter entirely to change a person's mind. The all-or-nothing dieter needs more than just a behavioural change—they need their minds changed, which is never easy.

Interestingly, I am pretty sure that I was an all-or-nothing dieter. Like Caroline, I had tried numerous diets, which came in handy as an obesity doctor. When patients came to see me to discuss their dieting history I knew firsthand about the programs they had tried. I was very well versed in every program, book, and herbal remedy available. I had spent thousands of dollars, hours, and tears on my next great dieting fix throughout my life, because the next program would finally be the one that would work. I would last a month or two at the most and then fall apart and rebound with a vengeance. Everything that had been denied to me for the previous month would now be on the menu in large quantities and at all times.

The following is by no means a scientifically proven test, but it is definitely a place to start to give you insight into your behaviour. Answer the following questions:

1. How often do you go on a new diet?
    a. Once a year
    b. Every three to four months
    c. Monthly
    d. Daily; tomorrow's the day

2. How long do you last on any given program?
    a. A while, then I fall off track but still retain some learning tools
    b. A month at the most
    c. About two to three months
    d. Sometimes I never start

3. How many diet books have you read or started to read in the last ten years?
   a. None
   b. One or two
   c. Three
   d. One a year (or more)

4. When you start a program do you have euphoria about the program and follow it with strict intensity?
   a. Not really. I'm pretty realistic about what I want.
   b. This new program is really interesting. I may learn something that will help me lose weight.
   c. I feel great starting something new.
   d. This program is going to be the one. This will finally fix what's wrong with me.

Look at the answers you gave to these questions. Is there a polarizing pattern to your dieting habits? Have you answered "d" to most of these questions? Understand that this is *not* a medical diagnosis but an exercise that gives you some insight into your patterns of behaviour. Still unsure where you stand? Consider these questions:

1. Do you create unrealistic expectations around diet and exercise?

   For example:
   a. Do you promise to work out every day even though you have not been exercising before?
   b. Do you swear you will never eat (insert name of food here) again? Even though you love that food?
   c. Do you set deadlines for weight loss that are physiologically unachievable?

2. When you start a diet, do you inappropriately adjust your current behaviour and environment to meet your new diet's needs?
   For example:
   a. You stop eating out.
   b. You bring your own food to parties and functions.
   c. You cancel or miss out on social gatherings to meet dieting needs.

3. Are you easily derailed from a program?
4. Once derailed from a program do you rebound with an "I don't care" attitude?
5. Do you look for opportunities to indulge in the foods that you have been "denied"?
6. Do you attach moral descriptors to certain foods such as "good" or "bad"?
7. When you are on a program, do you dwell on all the things you are giving up to diet?

If you answered "yes" to a majority of these questions you may have a pattern of weight management that is at either end of the spectrum: "all" or "nothing." Understand that some all-or-nothing dieters are really successful in their weight loss. What I mean is that they find the "all" and stick to it. I would argue that many people find a way to make the "all" stick. The issue, however, occurs when the fluctuation between these two extremes causes you to lose and gain weight repeatedly. Not only is this pendulum-swing approach to healthy eating hard on the body's metabolism and physiology, but it also eats away at a person's self-esteem.

When I first met Caroline she was almost visibly broken by her dieting history. She told me that starting another program right now would be like entering into a bad relationship. She explained, "I'm exhausted from the constant swinging back and forth. I feel like I build up a program, thinking this is the one, and then like a bad boyfriend it just let's me down. I lose the weight at first and then I watch myself, almost outside of myself, gaining it back, powerless to get back on the previous strict program that I was once on. It kills me. I want to lose weight but I just can't keep going through this back and forth." Caroline's story is common. It's this kind of yo-yo dieting experience that deflates people and discourages them from getting healthier. We are too often shaped more by our failures than our successes. Caroline focuses on the falls and not the climbs, and this has ruined her weight-management confidence. In short, she's lost her "dieting mojo."

Like Caroline, if you are an all-or-nothing dieter you probably have a tendency to polarize dieting into "good" or "bad," where you are either "behaving" or "cheating." But it's not about that. Health is actually a spectrum and not a series of on-and-off switches. When you spend your time polarizing your behaviour, you sit in judgment too often. This inevitably leads to an inability to learn from your behaviours. When you are too busy criticizing your mistakes you can't learn from them. Our journey to health is a process and not a series of divisions. We learn best when we can embrace our mistakes and use them as opportunities for improvement. So settle down with the diagnosis and the judgment and let's get to work with some strategies that may help you on the road ahead.

Picking the Right Game Plan

Step 1: Find Your Superpower

Most all-or-nothing dieters try to drastically change their patterns of behaviour immediately upon embarking on a diet. For them, a diet is like squeezing a square peg into a round hole. The key to changing this behaviour is to instead slowly sand the edges off the peg so that it eventually fits into the hole itself.

To do this effectively you have to pick a program that will fit into your current life. If you hate vegetables, going vegan is just plain stupid. If you have bad arthritis in both knees, then taking up running is ludicrous. You have to pick the best program for you that resembles certain life requirements based on where you struggle. Ask yourself the following questions:

1. Do I like structure or flexibility when it comes to choosing my food?
   a. Do I want a meal plan with everything laid out for me?
   b. Do I want to pick my own menu based on my daily likes and dislikes?
   c. Do I hate all this entirely and just want someone to prepare my meals for me?

2. Do I get bored with the same type of program?
   a. Do I need variety in my food choices and my exercise routine?
   b. How often do I want to switch things up?
   c. Do I need consistency in my food and exercise?

3. How can I plan for the inevitabilities of life?
   a. When I get derailed, how will I get back on track?
   b. Will I make sure that I retain one or two aspects of my new behaviour through the storm to make sure I come out the other side?

This group of Eating Personalities is notoriously good at finding a place to start. Sit down, ask yourself these questions, and begin. But understand that this time we are looking for the middle, not the end. We need to be honest with ourselves and use our past experience to help us see where the pitfalls happened. I don't want you to approach this with the idea "I can't do any programs because they don't work." Instead, I want you to look at what components of various programs and patterns of behaviour realistically fit into your life and can be modified. In short, figure out what your superpower is.

Caroline and I figured out that when she kept a food diary she was more conscious of her patterns of behaviour. She also notes that she loves keeping lists. Caroline's superpower is therefore her ability to keep a food diary. To find your superpower, ask yourself the following questions:

1. Am I good at keeping a log or a food diary?
2. Am I good at being consistent with my food choices?
3. Do I like following a set menu?
4. Do I like to prepare my own meals?
5. Do I like to be creative with my food choices and be in control?
6. Am I good at committing to an exercise program?

Which question did you answer "yes" to? That's your superpower. Caroline is great at food diaries. Me? I'm really consistent with my food choices. Stick me on a meal plan and I'm good to go. Many of my patients like following a set menu and therefore a menu plan is perfect for them. Others want flexibility and control and do very well coming up with their own plan and calorie counting. Find out what you're good at, and that is the first place to start.

Step 2: Find the Balance

Now that you know what your superpower is, you need to proceed with the next step. An all-or-nothing dieter has one of two options for their reform: They can either be all-or-something, or they can bring the two extreme poles together in a happy medium, perhaps more like a something-or-something dieter. This means taking the extremes of your behaviour and toning them down a bit.

Start with a food diary. Write down everything you eat for a few weeks. Regardless if this is not your strength, and even if you suck at a food diary, relax—you only need it as a starting point. If you are great at keeping a food diary then this will be a satisfying experience for you. Caroline had a food diary from her first month with me that looked something like the first one on the opposite page.

Caroline's Food Diary

	Sunday	Monday	Tuesday	Wednesday	Thursday	Friday	Saturday
Breakfast	French toast with syrup Large latte	Banana Cereal with milk	Scone Large latte	Oat fudge bar Large latte	Skipped	Scone Latte	Oat fudge bar Large latte
Lunch	???	Turkey sandwich Carrots, cucumbers, and dip	Chocolate bar	Granola bar Soup	Microwave popcorn	12 pieces of sushi Order of tempura	Burger and fries
Dinner	Lasagna Salad 2 chocolate chip cookies	Roasted chicken Baked potato Salad Brownie	Stir-fry Rice Brownie	Spaghetti (too much)	Rice Sweet potatoes Barbecued pork	Steak Baked potato	Birthday cake 3 pieces of pizza

	Sunday	Monday	Tuesday	Wednesday	Thursday	Friday	Saturday
Breakfast	French toast with syrup Large latte	Banana Cereal with milk	Scone Large latte	Oat fudge bar Large latte	Skipped	Scone Latte	Oat fudge bar Large latte
Lunch	???	Turkey sandwich Carrots, cucumbers, and dip	Chocolate bar	Granola bar Soup	Microwave popcorn	12 pieces of sushi Order of tempura	Burger and fries
Dinner	Lasagna Salad 2 chocolate chip cookies	Roasted chicken Baked potato Salad Brownie	Stir-fry Rice Brownie	Spaghetti (too much)	Rice Sweet potatoes Barbecued pork	Steak Baked potato	Birthday cake 3 pieces of pizza

Go through the food diary and circle the meals that could be made healthier, but start with one meal at a time. If we use the food diary from above you can see that I've chosen to "redecorate" breakfasts first. I'm taking advantage of the fact that Caroline's greatest strength is also her greatest hurdle—Caroline knows how to diet like nobody's business. As such, she is well versed in what she should be eating for a healthier diet and what she should avoid.

If you are like Caroline, highlight for yourself some alternatives that could be chosen instead of your previous breakfasts. In Caroline's case, her highlighted diary looks like the second one on page 77.

I've devoted an entire chapter in this book to meal makeover suggestions (see Chapter 11). For Caroline, however, the case is quite simple with her breakfasts: She needs to stop having dessert for breakfast. She is having scones or oat fudge bars for breakfast, both of which are pastries that are easily 500 calories or more. When she adds in a large latte her morning calorie count is now almost 800 calories. Her makeover is simple:

1. Sunday brunch as usual
2. Downsize the latte to a small made with low-fat milk
3. One pastry-based breakfast on Fridays
4. The remainder of the week she will choose a healthier breakfast from the list of better options below

Healthier breakfast options:

1. No-sugar cereal with low-fat milk and a piece of fruit
2. Oatmeal with a piece of fruit
3. Two slices of whole-wheat toast with peanut butter and a banana
4. Egg and egg white omelet with spinach, mushrooms, and low-fat cheese

Take a month to solidify your healthy changes and then move on to lunches. Again, take a month to solidify your healthy changes and then move on to dinners, snacks, and so on. Over the course of a six-month period you'll have successfully changed what you are eating and the timing is slow enough so that you are neither deprived nor denied.

It took Caroline almost eight months to remodel her meals. The best part of this slow process is that for an all-or-nothing dieter, constancy is the key. I pointed out that, for Caroline, this was essentially her longest, healthiest dieting relationship (if you could call it a diet). Make no mistake—Caroline still has her moments when her meals look like she has gone off track. The key here is that I'm trying to get Caroline to have indulgent meals *sometimes*, but not let them derail her.

The key with the all-or-nothing dieter is when they do fall off track, they need to minimize the fall and get back on track almost immediately. As I tell Caroline repeatedly:

You can have bad days, you just can't have bad weeks or months. Furthermore, the ultimate goal here is to turn those bad days into just bad meals. Don't let indulgent meals minimize all the good work you are doing. Always reflect on the positive changes you are making and don't focus on the less healthy choices.

Cheat Days

Let's talk about so-called "cheat days." This is a conventional mode of allowing people on a diet to indulge on a specific day and have all the foods they are missing out on during the week of dieting. I have read claims suggesting that the body does better during these times because the brain does not feel deprived, which will allow for even better weight loss.

I am not a fan of cheat days. First of all, cheat days imply a sense of deviance that I think is rather unhealthy in principle. You are all grown men and women; this is not grade school and it's not a test. If you want to have a burger and fries, have it. Eat it responsibly, eyes wide open, and ensure that your other meals for the day are healthy. Go for an extra walk that day, and think of this as a treat in an otherwise healthy lifestyle. Cheat days promote the idea that if you are strict six days a week you can be a nutritional lunatic on Saturdays or Sundays. It promotes the idea of binge eating, which is a dangerous message to the all-or-nothing dieter and to anyone trying to make a healthy change. I take a different approach with my patients: I advocate designated treats. Make a list of your five favourite treats; Caroline's list looked like this:

- Brownie
- Oat fudge bar
- Chocolate chip cookies
- Ice cream
- Movie popcorn

We then incorporated these treats into her weekly diet for two weeks. The only rules she had were that she could not have two treats on the same day, she had to ensure that her other meals were healthy with plenty of vegetables and fruit, and she had to exercise a bare minimum of thirty minutes per day.

With this in mind, Caroline's food diary looked something like the table on the next page, with her treats highlighted.

Over the next month she had to eliminate one of the treats each week. The following month Caroline was down to three treats a week. Her new food rules stipulated that she could have at least three treats a week and a maximum of five per week. Every couple of months she was instructed to revisit this issue and see how she was doing. After eight months, Caroline's food diary showed significant signs of improvement. Caroline had found a balance, which was her key. See for yourself on page 82.

The plan of attack with a person who diets and indulges in extremes really is to find the balance in the everyday. That being said, the next plan of attack is to navigate the times when the

Caroline's Food Diary Including Treats

	Sunday	Monday	Tuesday	Wednesday	Thursday	Friday	Saturday
Breakfast	Banana Cereal with milk	Banana Cereal with milk	Banana Cereal with milk	Oat fudge bar Small latte	Skipped	Banana Cereal with milk	Oat fudge bar Large latte
Lunch	Movie popcorn	Turkey sandwich Carrots, cucumbers, and dip	Protein bar Apple	Granola bar Soup Apple	Lean Cuisine	12 pieces of sushi Chocolate chip cookie from a bakery	Burger Salad
Dinner	Lasagna Salad	Roasted chicken Baked potato Salad Brownie	Stir-fry Rice Brownie	Spaghetti (too much)	Sweet potatoes Barbecued pork Ice cream cone	Steak Baked potato	Pizza Salad

Caroline's Balanced Food Diary

	Sunday	Monday	Tuesday	Wednesday	Thursday	Friday	Saturday
Breakfast	French toast with syrup Large latte	Banana Cereal with milk Coffee	Banana Cereal with milk Coffee	Banana Cereal with milk Coffee	Oat fudge bar Coffee	Banana Cereal with milk Coffee	Egg white omelet Coffee
Lunch	???	Turkey sandwich Carrots, cucumbers, and dip	Protein bar Yogurt Fruit	Granola bar Soup Apple	Lean Cuisine 2 tangerines	12 pieces of sushi	Burger and fries
Dinner	Lasagna Salad 2 chocolate chip cookies	Roasted chicken Baked potato	Stir-fry Rice Brownie	Homemade chili Salad	Sweet potatoes Barbecued pork	Steak Baked potato	2 pieces of pizza Salad

balance is disrupted (as it always will be) when life throws us all little reminders about its uncertainty. Sure, it's rather unfortunate to have unpredictability and uncertainty around every corner, but doesn't that just make us all a little better at problem solving?

Step 3: Forgive and Move On

I would argue that I learned more in life from my mistakes than from my achievements. Sure, it is not nearly as enjoyable an educational experience, but it is more significant. As a doctor, my profession demands perfection. As a person, I'm a human being that cannot always deliver. Sometimes I make mistakes, both in my work and in my life. The important thing is to acknowledge the error and move on. When we recognize our mistakes we can learn from them. It's important to accept that you are a person and by your very nature you will learn by mistake. The key is to acknowledge, forgive, and move on. With patients, I apologize. I recognize my mistake (or it is made clear for me) and try not to do it again. In my everyday life, I try to navigate away from places and situations that have been harmful in the past to avoid mistakes once made.

I will give you some specific strategies about avoiding mistakes in Chapter 13, which focuses on getting back on track, but in the meantime accept that life will happen. If you give up every time things don't go the way you planned, you are done before you even begin. Come to this process from a positive place and a place of forgiveness and you will open up a classroom that you never dreamed existed.

7

The Portion Distorter

There is a unique group of overweight and obese patients that I see on a daily basis. This group is nutritionally sound and quite diet savvy—they know how to eat healthy, and they know what they should and should not eat. If you were to search through their kitchens and their pantries right now you would find a pretty respectable list of goods: plenty of fruits and vegetables and a well-rounded nutritional platform. Many of these people might consider themselves bona fide "foodies." They don't eat fast food and they never drink pop or fruit juice. They might be emotional eaters, but only as they really enjoy food. They are committed to healthy nutritional eating. They are, however, overweight or obese. This group of people eats well by all nutritional standards but, plain and simple, they eat too much.

I first met Stephanie in 2009 when her family doctor referred her to me. If I were not Stephanie's doctor, I'd probably have her as a friend; she is a delight. Stephanie is a full-time mother of three girls. She shops exclusively at Whole Foods and predominately eats organic. Her daughters have never seen the inside of a McDonald's restaurant and if Stephanie has a say, they never will.

Meals in Stephanie's home are out of a magazine. Stephanie loves to cook. She uses local products whenever possible and even bakes her own bread from scratch. She gets up and makes breakfast every morning for the family. She prepares whole-grain pancakes from scratch, Italian frittatas, egg-white scrambles, or homemade granola and yogurt. She uses olive oil to cook with and there is always an abundance of fresh fruit in her house. Stephanie drives her girls to school, handing them their homemade lunches, and then drives home to begin her day, which will involve planning dinner for that night.

Stephanie is baffled by her weight problem. She gained about twenty to thirty pounds with each pregnancy and found it a challenge to lose the weight after the baby was born. As Stephanie tells me, "I never eat fast food, I don't drink crap. We eat really well, so what is my problem?"

Stephanie's issues go beyond her food and activity levels. I am convinced there is a significant amount of body–brain chemistry that is contributing to her weight problem. I don't think Stephanie's problem is purely her behaviour. In fact, I think much of her inability to lose weight may stem from her own biochemistry and her genetic makeup. I am also convinced that Stephanie and many like her don't realize how truly challenging lifelong weight loss can be. What Stephanie thinks she has to do to lose weight and what she really has to do to lose weight permanently are two entirely different things.

There may very well be a huge component of Stephanie's weight problem that is due to her body chemistry and genetics. We will likely never know; modern medicine has yet to make such strides in obesity medicine. At this point in time, where Stephanie is concerned, all we have to work on is her behaviour. Furthermore, improving Stephanie's behaviour toward food will benefit her overall health.

Stephanie honestly has no idea where she is going wrong. In her mind, she is following all the rules: She eats most of her meals at home and they really are nutritious; she cooks a healthy Mediterranean-based diet; she never drinks her calories; she eats breakfast every morning and has not seen the inside of a fast-food joint since the early 80s. I feel for Stephanie, because her frustration is so common. Most of us have no idea what it takes to lose weight, keep it off, and maintain a healthier life. Most of us don't realize how much of a challenge this pursuit can be.

Stephanie is baffled to explain her slow weight gain. She feels she is more active now than she was in her twenties, and her eating patterns have been established for the past thirty years. Much to her surprise, though, Stephanie did not have to change anything to gain weight. As Stephanie's body ages, she needs less food and her environment has not changed to accommodate this. If anything, Stephanie is eating more now than ever and she doesn't even realize it.

Stephanie is a portion distorter. Interestingly, she has a great deal of company; North Americans are pretty good at this game of portion distortion. We need visual cues to let us know how much we have eaten, since we can't rely solely on our stomachs to tell our brains when we are full. A study using self-refilling food bowls proved this point quite nicely.[45] The study, published in *Obesity Research* in 2005, recruited fifty-four participants of various body sizes and separated them randomly into two different groups. The first group was given a normal bowl of soup and told to eat the entire bowl. The second group of participants was given a bowl of soup that continuously refilled itself. Both bowls were housed in a particular apparatus so that the soup eaters did not know that their bowls were being refilled. Furthermore, the bowls were refilled very slowly so that the soup eaters did not realize they were eating a bottomless bowl until some time had passed.

Participants who were eating from a bottomless soup bowl ate 73 percent more soup than those who ate from a regular soup bowl. What was even more surprising was that those with endless soup bowls did not realize that they had eaten more than their "regular bowl" counterparts, nor did they feel fuller or more sated than those who had consumed just a regular bowl of soup. These results were independent of body mass index.

Portion size has in fact doubled over the last thirty years. And it's not just the amount of food we put on our plates. Our food units themselves have gotten bigger over the last three decades. For instance, I came of age during this country's first muffin craze. I remember the first coffee shops coming out with muffins for sale and being able to buy them in the grocery store en masse. This was back in the 1970s. A muffin in 1980 was 1.5 ounces (40 grams) and had 210 calories. Today the average muffin is 4 ounces (115 grams) and 500 calories. To burn off just the difference between yesterday's muffin and today's muffin you would have to run for thirty minutes.[46] The same is true if we go back to my favourite past-time snack: a package of movie licorice. Back in 1979 the movie licorice that I bought was 200 grams and about 700 calories. Today the average movie licorice package is easily twice that size.

According to the 2007 Canadian Community Health Survey we really are eating more of everything. The survey looked at household consumption between 1970 and 2004 and found significant increases in the amounts of grains, refined sugars, and fats we are eating.[47] Take a look:

Increase in Annual Household Consumption of Different Food Groups from 1970 to 2004

Nutrient	Annual consumption per household in 1970 (in pounds)	Annual consumption per household in 2004 (in pounds)	% increase in consumption (rounded up)
Grains	136	200	47
Refined sugars	139	172	24
Protein	588	621	6
Fruits	241	280	16
Vegetables	337	425	26
Fats	56	77	38

I would argue that a big part of this increased consumption has to do with an increase in the sizes of the things we eat every day. If we take a closer look at then-and-now portion sizes we see something really striking: The sizes of our staples that we eat every day are larger than they used to be.[48]

How Much Have Our Staple Foods Changed in Size and Calories?

Item	Size and calories in 1980	Size and calories today
Coffee	Regular with cream and sugar 45 calories	Grande mocha with whipped cream 400 calories
Bagel	3 inches in diameter 140 calories	6 inches in diameter 350 calories
Muffin	1.5 ounces 210 calories	4 ounces 500 calories
Chicken Caesar salad	1.5 cups 390 calories	3.5 cups 790 calories
Chicken stir-fry	2 cups 435 calories	4.5 cups 865 calories
Chocolate chip cookie	1.5 inches in diameter 55 calories	4.5 inches in diameter 275 calories
Movie popcorn	5 cups 210 calories	11 cups 630 calories
French fries	2.4 ounces 210 calories	6.9 ounces 610 calories
Cheeseburger	330 calories	590 calories
Spaghetti with meatballs	1 cup with sauce and 3 small meatballs 500 calories	2 cups with sauce and 3 large meatballs 1025 calories
Pop	1.5 ounces 85 calories	20 ounces 250 calories

As you can see, there is a great disparity between the sizes of the foods we eat every day and the sizes of the foods we eat on special occasions; movie theatre popcorn has grown as much as bagels and muffins.

When Stephanie tells me that her food choices have not changed in thirty years but her weight has, she's really not far off. Not only has her metabolism altered as she aged, but more importantly Stephanie is eating more than she thinks she is. It really does not matter that Stephanie eats as well as she did thirty years ago. If we do the math, in reality she is eating double what she used to eat without even trying.

Stephanie's road to restructuring her portions begins with the same strategy most of my patients begin with—a food diary. It really does help patients see what they are doing, eyes wide open. Stephanie's food diary needs one additional detail, though. I ask her to measure all her food for one week. I don't ask her to make any changes to what she is currently eating. Instead I want her to take her usual portion sizes and measure them to find out how much she is eating. Everything gets measured: cereals for breakfast, peanut butter on her toast, mayonnaise and salad dressings, rice and potatoes. I also ask Stephanie to weigh her proteins for one week. Her one-week food diary looked something like the one on the next spread.

As you can see from Stephanie's meal plan she does eat well. She only eats out once a week and does not drink her calories. The issue with Stephanie's eating behaviour is that her portion sizes are much larger than they need to be. Furthermore, Stephanie's food diary shows that she eats a lot of extras in the way of oils and dressings and spreads. Stephanie and I sit down and figure out where she could trim her portion sizes, meal by meal. We begin with Stephanie's breakfasts.

First I suggest that Stephanie switch her cream to milk. She'll cut out 100 calories per day, or 700 calories per week, with one simple change. The other thing that we discuss is if Stephanie could either go to one piece of toast per day or if she could cut back on the size of her Saturday omelet. Stephanie decides that she wants two pieces of toast per day, but she can easily switch to milk and cut her Saturday omelet in half and only have one piece of toast on that

Stephanie's Food Diary

Sunday	Monday	Tuesday	Wednesday	Thursday	Friday	Saturday
2 pieces of French toast 2 tbsp maple syrup 2 cups coffee with 4 tbsp of cream	2 pieces of whole-grain toast with 2 tbsp of peanut butter Banana 2 cups of coffee with 4 tbsp of cream	2 pieces of whole-grain toast with 2 tbsp of peanut butter Banana 2 cups of coffee with 4 tbsp of cream	2 pieces of whole-grain toast with 2 tbsp of peanut butter Banana 2 cups of coffee with 4 tbsp of cream	2 pieces of whole-grain toast with 2 tbsp of peanut butter Banana 2 cups of coffee with 4 tbsp of cream	2 pieces of whole-grain toast with 2 tbsp of peanut butter Banana 2 cups of coffee with 4 tbsp of cream	3-egg omelet with 1 cup spinach, 1 tbsp olive oil, 3 ounces of cheese 2 pieces of whole-grain toast with 2 tsp of butter 2 cups of coffee with 4 tbsp of cream
6 ounces of tofu 2 cups of vegetables 2 tbsp of olive oil 1 cup of brown rice	Greek salad with 4 ounces of feta, 3 cups of vegetables, 20 olives, and 2 tbsp of olive oil 1 piece of pita 3 tbsp of hummus	Greek salad with 4 ounces of feta, 3 cups of vegetables, 20 olives, and 2 tbsp of olive oil 1 piece of pita 3 tbsp of hummus	2 cups of vegetarian chili made with 8 ounces of tofu, lots of veggies, 3 tbsp of tomato paste, 1 can of tomatoes, 1 cup of black beans 1/2 avocado 1 flour tortilla	2 cups of vegetarian chili made with 8 ounces of tofu, lots of veggies, 3 tbsp of tomato paste, 1 can of tomatoes, 1 cup of black beans 1/2 avocado 1 flour tortilla	8 ounces of chicken breast 1 cup of sweet potatoes 1 cup of beets roasted with 1 tbsp olive oil 2 cups of salad with 1 tbsp olive oil and balsamic vinegar	6 ounces of tofu 2 cups of vegetables 2 tbsp of olive oil 1 cup of brown rice

Sunday	Monday	Tuesday	Wednesday	Thursday	Friday	Saturday
8 ounces of chicken breast 1 cup of sweet potatoes 1 cup of beets roasted with 1 tbsp olive oil 2 cups of salad with 1 tbsp olive oil and balsamic vinegar	2 cups of home-made chili with lean ground beef, vegetables, and beans 1 apple	2 flour tortillas 6 ounces of chicken 2 cups peppers and tomatoes 1/4 cup sour cream 1/4 cup salsa 1 banana	6 ounces of tofu 2 cups of vegetables 2 tbsp olive oil 1 cup of brown rice 1 orange	6 ounces pork chop 1 cup of sweet potatoes 1 cup of beets roasted with 1 tbsp olive oil 2 cups of salad with 1 tbsp olive oil and balsamic vinegar	2 flour tortillas 6 ounces of chicken 2 cups peppers and tomatoes 1/4 cup sour cream 1/4 cup salsa	8 ounces of grilled salmon 1 baked potato with 3 tbsp of sour cream Salad with 3 tbsp of dressing 1 piece of apple pie 2 glasses of wine

day. She's sticking with her French toast on Sunday, too—it is her special brunch, after all.

Blueprint for Change

The lesson we can learn from Stephanie is how to use a food diary as a blueprint for change. She looks at what she's doing and sees where she can budget. The key with a portion distorter is a three-step process:

1. Look for hidden calories
2. Put your plate on a budget
3. Do a food audit

Step 1: Look for Hidden Calories

Many portion distorters have a significant amount of their calories coming from sauces, oils, and spreads. I call these "hidden calories." The key here is to modify the condiments. I suggest to Stephanie that she use either non-fat cooking spray or chicken broth to cook her food, or even to put her olive oil in a spray bottle and spray the pan with it. Here's the exercise: Look at how you prepare your food and look at what you're putting on your food. Chances are these items can be modified. See the chart at the top of the next page.

In addition to remodelling her hidden calories, Stephanie needs to re-examine her portion sizes to see where she can cut back on the size or amount of the things she eats.

Old item	New item	Calories saved
2 tbsp of olive oil (180 calories)	Low-fat cooking spray or using a spray bottle to spray olive oil on the pan (2–30 calories)	150–178 calories
2 tbsp regular salad dressing (average type) (140 calories)	2 tbsp low-fat salad dressing or fat-free salad dressing (30–60 calories)	80–110 calories
4 tbsp teriyaki sauce (120 calories)	Low-sodium soy sauce (4 calories)	116 calories
4 tbsp guacamole (120 calories)	4 tbsp salsa (40 calories)	80 calories
2 tbsp maple syruup (104 calories)	1/2 cup fresh fruit (50 calories)	56 calories
2 tbsp jam (208 calories)	1/2 banana (45 calories)	163 calories
2 tbsp mayonnaise (115 calories)	Mustard (5 calories) or Greek yogurt (40 calories)	75–110 calories

Step 2: Put Your Plate on a Budget

Let's take Stephanie's lunches as the perfect place to put her plate on a budget (see page 94).

I ask Stephanie to cut her portions by 25–50 percent for one month and to institute some of the adjustments to her hidden calories that I mentioned above. She doesn't need to make any adjustments to her vegetables. This means that, in theory, her diary in one month's time will look like the one on page 95.

The lesson Stephanie teaches us is that portion sizes are a sneaky thing. They need to be changed over time. Furthermore, I recommend to my patients to modify slowly—no more than one meal per month. Take a month to modify breakfasts, then a month for lunches, and so on.

The final step for the portion distorter is to ensure that these changes stick. You don't need to measure your portions for the rest of your life, but a food audit is a very good idea.

Old Lunches

Sunday	Monday	Tuesday	Wednesday	Thursday	Friday	Saturday
6 ounces of tofu 2 cups of vegetables 2 tbsp of olive oil 1 cup of brown rice	Greek salad with 4 ounces of feta, 3 cups of vegetables, 20 olives, and 2 tbsp of olive oil 1 piece of pita 3 tbsp of hummus	Greek salad with 4 ounces of feta, 3 cups of vegetables, 20 olives, and 2 tbsp of olive oil 1 piece of pita 3 tbsp of hummus	2 cups of vegetarian chili made with 8 ounces of tofu, lots of veggies, 3 tbsp of tomato paste, 1 can of tomatoes, 1 cup of black beans 1/2 avocado 1 flour tortilla	2 cups of vegetarian chili made with 8 ounces of tofu, lots of veggies, 3 tbsp of tomato paste, 1 can of tomatoes, 1 cup of black beans 1/2 avocado 1 flour tortilla	8 ounces of chicken breast 1 cup of sweet potatoes 1 cup of beets roasted with 1 tbsp olive oil 2 cups of salad with 1 tbsp olive oil and balsamic vinegar	6 ounces of tofu 2 cups of vegetables 2 tbsp of olive oil 1 cup of brown rice

Lunches "On a Budget"

Sunday	Monday	Tuesday	Wednesday	Thursday	Friday	Saturday
4 ounces of tofu 2 cups of vegetables 2 sprays of olive oil 2/3 cup of brown rice	Greek salad with 3 ounces of feta, 3 cups of vegetables, 13 olives, and 1 tbsp of olive oil 1/2 piece of pita 2 tbsp of hummus	Greek salad with 3 ounces of feta, 3 cups of vegetables, 13 olives, 1 tbsp of olive oil 1/2 piece of pita 2 tbsp of hummus	1.5 cups of vegetarian chili made with 6 ounces of tofu, lots of veggies, 3 tbsp of tomato paste, 1 can of tomatoes, 1 cup of black beans 1/4 avocado 1/2 flour tortilla	1.5 cups of vegetarian chili made with 6 ounces of tofu, lots of veggies, 3 tbsp of tomato paste, 1 can of tomatoes, 1 cup of black beans 1/4 avocado 1/2 flour tortilla	5 ounces of chicken breast 1/2 cup of sweet potatoes 1 cup of beets roasted with 1/2 tbsp olive oil 2 cups of salad with 1/2 tbsp olive oil and balsamic vinegar	4 ounces of tofu 2 cups of vegetables Non-fat cooking spray 3/4 cup of brown rice

Step 3: Do a Regular Food Audit

Doing a food audit means spending a week keeping a food diary and measuring everything you put in your mouth. This allows you to see if your portion sizes are going back to their previous size. Remember that you live in a world that does not give you a proper frame of reference—portion sizes are twice what they used to be. If you don't do a food audit every few months you will lull yourself back into a false sense of portion security.

The final lesson here is that this process, like all others, needs constant attention. You may find as you progress through these changes that you only need to audit yourself every few months or every few weeks. Or you may find that you need to weigh and measure foods one day each week; I have many patients who pick one day every week when they weigh and measure their food. Other patients prefer to take one week every month or two and use that as the week to audit their behaviour and portion sizes. I leave it up to you. Remember that the key here is to keep an open mind—use your behaviour as a learning tool. If you find that a weekly audit every few months is not enough, then change the frequency. Work within your own limitations and learn from them what your capacity for change is.

8

The Sitting Duck

Meet Elaine. She is fifty-six years old, hates exercise, and her idea of a relaxing evening is coming home from work, eating dinner, and spending the night reading a book with a glass of wine. Elaine's kids have all grown and left home, and she and her husband now have a ritual: They sit together after dinner with the music playing and they read. They go through books by the shelf-full. Elaine has a treadmill that she bought when her youngest son moved out; it sits in his old room that she has turned into an office. Her husband uses it faithfully, getting on it every night as he watches the evening news. Elaine pours herself a glass of wine and prepares dinner. Elaine loves to cook.

By day, Elaine works in an office. She gets up at about 7 A.M. and gets ready for work. She eats breakfast at home, then drives to work, stopping on the way at the drive-through coffee shop for her morning fuel. At work during the day she sits at a desk. She tells me that there are times when she is asked to deliver papers to another floor in the office, so she gets up from her desk, goes to the elevator, and makes her way to whatever floor is required. Elaine gets an hour for lunch, but often eats her bagged lunch at her desk or buys a sandwich from a nearby deli. In the summer she will sit outside in the courtyard across from the office building and eat her lunch in the sunshine.

Elaine is fifty pounds overweight. A year ago she was diagnosed with hypertension, and her most recent blood work has shown that she has impaired fasting blood sugar, or borderline diabetes. Elaine's father died of a heart attack at the age of fifty-two; her older brother is sixty years old and he just had angioplasty; all of Elaine's mother's family has type 2 diabetes. Elaine is scared shitless.

Elaine is obviously nervous as she sits in my office at our first meeting. She is terrified that I am going to make her conform to unrealistic demands. She does not want to lose her life's rituals, but she also does not want to lose out on a healthy future. She perceives her family history as a bit of a self-fulfilling prophecy, but she is nonetheless determined to do something about it.

Elaine's biggest issue, from a cardiovascular risk perspective, is that she is what I call a sitting duck. Let's be clear—I don't want Elaine to exercise just to lose weight. In fact, I would argue that Elaine can't lose weight with exercise alone. My biggest issue with Elaine is that she really needs to exercise to reduce her risk of heart disease, stroke, and cancer. There are numerous studies in the medical and scientific literature that confirm this. What many people don't realize is that the medical literature shows a significant benefit just from walking compared to a sedentary lifestyle.[49] For example, examination of the Women's Health Initiative Observation Study looked at the health benefits of walking in preventing heart attacks and strokes.[50] The study looked at 73,743 women from fifty to seventy-nine years of age and compared the amount of time they spent walking along with their walking speeds with their rates of heart attack and stroke. These rates were compared with the cardiovascular rates of women who were sedentary. Women who walked more than a hundred minutes per week had a 29–63 percent reduction in their risk of heart attack and stroke compared to women who did not. The numbers vary based on the speed the women walked—the faster the walker, the lower the risk.

The thing that fascinates me about this study in particular is that it shows what we call a "dose response" to exercise. In medicine we see this response with certain medications: the higher the dose of the medication, the higher the response. In this hallmark trial, we see that the higher the dose of exercise, the greater the cardiovascular response. That being said, even the slowest walkers saw a benefit, which of course reinforces my belief that something is something, and it's certainly better than nothing.

Exercise for Your Health, Not Your Waistline

Yes, exercise does decrease your overall risk of heart disease. Further, studies show that exercise lowers a person's risk of developing diabetes, hypertension, and certain cancers. But contrary to popular belief, exercise alone is a terrible way to lose weight.[51, 52]

Let me give you a couple of examples. In February 2011, I climbed Mount Kilimanjaro, which is the highest free-standing peak in the world, standing at 5895 metres above sea level. I was turning forty and needed a grand gesture, and climbing this monstrosity seemed like an excellent pursuit of both madness and greatness all on one endeavour. I spent ten days climbing Kili, and I lost five pounds. In the summer of that same year my husband and I cycled across Canada in a relay to raise money for type 2 diabetes. We got on our bikes in Vancouver on August 13 and rode a hundred kilometres every day for twenty-one days. After cycling 2156 kilometres in total I stepped on the scale—I was down eight pounds. Sure my odometer said I had burned over 5000 calories a day, but I knew that was wrong.

My body was designed to conserve its energy, so there was no way my hips were giving it up that easily. Furthermore, I had spent a lifetime convincing my brain through one diet after another that it was starving. There was no physiological reality where my fat tissue was just going to "give up the ghost" and get lost. Remember, our evolutionary DNA has spent hundreds of thousands of years evolving to adapt to periods of starvation and the fact that we, not so long ago, used to run down our food. It has only been in the last half century or so that obtaining food became a rather low-intensity experience.

The first reason why exercise alone is the worst way to lose weight is that we were designed to run down our food—literally. Five hundred years ago when our ancestors wanted a snack they had to go outside and catch it or harvest it. If I was living in Canada in the 1500s and I wanted dinner, I had to wait for the buffalo run or the salmon run or some sort of animal to run by. Then I had to chase it down, kill it, clean it, and prepare it for cooking. I then had to chop down a tree, build a fire, and roast whatever I had killed for dinner.

Fast-forward to the early 1900s and I was still working pretty hard for my food. Maybe I had a farm on the prairies that grew grain or potatoes. I had to work the field all day and when harvest time came around I could pick my grain, sheave it by hand, grind it, and make it into flour that could then be made (by hand) into bread. I built my own fire and baked my own bread or boiled my potatoes.

In either case, by the time I had made my meal I had burnt more calories than was in the meal itself. Our bodies have spent thousands of years adapting to the fact that we had to expend a significant amount of energy to attain and prepare our food. Furthermore, food was not always plentiful. Famine is far more prevalent in our history than are times of feast. As such, humans have evolved to adapt to times of famine quite well.[53] Given this, when we do start to exercise our bodies automatically begin working at all costs to conserve energy. Think about it: If you are designed to run down food, you are going to do everything you can to conserve energy while running down that food.

Studies show that within four weeks of starting an exercise program you will begin to conserve energy. What does this mean? Step on the treadmill and plug in your age and weight on the machine's display. After an hour it will tell you that you burned a certain number of calories in that hour. If you've been active for more than a month, take that amount of calories and subtract about a third of it, because your body has adapted to your level of exercise.[54]

If you want to lose weight by exercise alone, stop right there. Without some sort of dietary therapy, exercise alone (at least the type of exercise most people would do in this situation) contributes very little to weight loss. Don't take my word for it—several clinical trials have been published that address this point.[55] In these trials the investigators took two groups of predominantly overweight men. They asked them to engage in a program of moderate-intensity physical activity four days a week for one year. The weight loss in these groups was measured after a year and compared to a "control group" of men who were relatively sedentary.[56] The moderate-intensity physical activity was essentially brisk walking on a treadmill at 4.0 miles per hour for about forty-five to sixty minutes at a time four days a week (or the equivalent). In the seven studies of this nature, the men who exercised regularly lost about two kilograms (four-and-a-half pounds) on average. Moreover, it's not known in these studies if the "exercise group" actually did modify their food intake because they were enrolled in an exercise program. There are also studies looking at vigorous-intensity exercise in obese people that show that daily vigorous exercise for more than sixty to ninety minutes at a time contributes to much more significant weight loss in this population.[57]

Exercise is a bit of a tricky thing with weight loss. Some dietary programs actually advocate that their participants *not* exercise while enrolled in their programs. There is a small contingent in certain medical circles that believe exercise increases hunger hormones. However, several studies have shown that this is not the case. A variety of trials have looked at hunger hormone levels and the experience of hunger post-exercise, particularly among lean individuals, and have found no increase in hunger or in food intake after exercise.[58]

However, one study published in the *American Journal of Clinical Nutrition* in 1990 showed that non-obese women who exercised experienced an immediate decrease in food intake immediately after exercise.[59] Obese women did not experience any change in food intake after exercise compared to their non-obese counterparts. I can see how this lack of change in food intake, namely this failure to decrease appetite, might be misinterpreted as an increase in food intake but again, the science shoots that idea down.

I suspect the debate will continue, and unfortunately it may dissuade some people from taking up exercise. Increased hunger or not, the cardiovascular benefits of even modest amounts of exercise are huge. Furthermore, as we explore below, when we do exercise while we are losing weight it prevents fat-free mass loss, which is the lean body tissue (muscle) you lose in addition to fat when you lose weight. Remember that muscle tissue burns far more energy than fat tissue does, so maintaining or increasing our muscle tissue through exercise is important.

Our bodies all have a resting energy expenditure, or REE. This is the amount of energy we need just to keep our heart beating, lungs breathing, and brain working. It is what is commonly called our "metabolism," but it is so much more than that term implies. Every tissue we have plays a role in your body's resting energy expenditure. Muscle tissue accounts for about 20 percent of your body's total REE. It stands to reason that the more muscle mass you have, the more energy you will require to keep it going. Fat tissue, on the other hand, accounts for about 2 percent of our bodies' REE.[60]

When we lose weight we lose both muscle *and* fat. About 75 percent of the weight we lose when we engage in any diet is from fat and 25 percent is from fat-free mass (FFM), which is mostly muscle. By adding physical activity to any program you reduce that fat-free mass loss to about 10 percent.

Two large-scale trials looked at this very phenomenon. They pooled data from forty-six and twenty-eight trials, respectively, and found that when exercise is added to any weight-loss program it will minimize FFM loss.[61] One study looked at people with a mean weight loss of ten kilograms (about twenty-two pounds); exercise dropped the loss of FFM in half. In men the rate of loss dropped from 28 percent to 13 percent; in women the rate of FFM loss dropped from 24 to 11 percent.[62]

Getting Your Head in the Game

One of the biggest changes I see in my practice with people exercising is the role it plays on their headspace. Let's be clear: Changing what you eat even when it is proactive and positive is still about what you can't have and what you can't do. I see it every day. We mourn the loss of ice cream and sweets, of lavish dinners out and lazy days on the couch. Part of this is because for many of us food was really enjoyable—it was a best friend. When we make any change to this pattern of eating we can't help but focus on what we've lost. I will address this "loss" in upcoming chapters, but for now what's important to note is that exercise *gives* us an added sense of accomplishment throughout this process. We start slowly and see what our bodies can do. We watch our fitness improve in a few short weeks, and it is remarkable to see how we were really made to move.

Let's go back to Elaine. Elaine just does not like to exercise, and her idea of a relaxing evening is sitting with a book—it is not going out for a walk. Elaine makes me think about the reasons why many of us don't move more. Here's a list of the most popular statements I've heard in my career regarding why my patients don't exercise:

1. I don't like to exercise.
2. I find exercise really boring.
3. Exercise hurts. I don't like to get all sweaty and short of breath. It's not comfortable.
4. I have arthritis in my knees/hips/back and can't move well.
5. I have no time to exercise.

6. I'm too tired to exercise. I come home from work at the end of the day and by the time I'm finished with the kids and the dinner and the household chores I'm exhausted.
7. I'm embarrassed to go to a gym or a pool.
8. I don't even know where to start.

So let's tackle the list and give you some strategies to get you moving more in spite of your reasons not to.

Reason #1: I Don't Like to Exercise

Guess what? Me neither. People are shocked when they hear that. I have never loved running, yet I've run marathons and half marathons. I don't mind swimming, but there are days when I just don't have it in me. I bike to work every day, but I must admit there are many times when I would love to take a cab instead.

I've been physically active every day for over a decade and I'm still waiting for what people call the "runner's high." Sure there are times when I'm on a beautiful bike ride and the sun is out and the air is perfect and I feel like I could ride forever. But these days happen maybe once every thirty rides. They are not often enough to keep me going. I don't exercise because I like exercise; I exercise because I can.

People who don't like exercise have one of three options:

1. Continue to hate exercise and don't do it
2. Continue to hate exercise but do it anyway
3. Do something you love along with something you hate. In other words, water down the hate for exercise by focusing on something else while you do it.

Reason #2: I Find Exercise Really Boring

I hear you. But there can be certain activities that are interesting. Some of this involves trying different things and seeing what interests you. Here's an exercise: Make a list of the things you enjoy doing and try to find some physically based activities around that. This point builds on one of the suggestions in Reason #1: Do something you love with something you hate. If you like spending time outdoors then a gym is the worst place for you; go for a walk instead. If you love watching television, get a piece of exercise equipment and put it in front of a television set. You need to amuse yourself while you exercise as a distraction. Here are some ideas to start you on the right track:

1. Join a walking group or make your own; having someone to talk to is a great way to ease the boredom.
2. A television and a treadmill is a powerful pairing; pick your favourite show and make that the time you exercise.
3. Listen to a book on tape while you exercise.
4. Join a team sport.
5. There are plenty of boot camps or exercise classes specifically geared toward beginners or people with weight issues. Why not give one a try?

Reason #3: Exercise Hurts

Yes, it does. But it won't always be that way. Sure sometimes we have to do things that are not easy. Most things in life don't come easy for any of us. The interesting thing about exercise is that everyone gets better at it regardless of where they start.

I learned to ride a bike when I was a kid. It had a classic 1970s banana seat bicycle and I loved it. It had streamers on the handlebars and a big bell. I can remember being a kid and riding my bike every summer night in the street until it got dark and my mom would flash the porch lights for us to come in and go to bed. Do you remember when you were a kid and exercise was play? We would run in the streets and play baseball or hockey or soccer or whatever. Exercise wasn't work—it was fun. And then we got old and life took over and exercise lost its play. Now it is all about work. So I propose we bring back the play.

When I bought my first racing bike I was not a cyclist. Truthfully, I had not owned a decent bike in years. I walked into a cycle shop in Vancouver and picked my first racing bike based on its colour alone. I knew nothing about bikes, but I knew that I loved riding a bike as a kid and it was time to bring back the play. Now, five years later, I don't own a car but I have three bicycles and I love them all even more than my first banana seat bike.

Find the sport you loved as a kid and modify it to meet your daily needs now. Sure it will be hard at first, but eventually you'll get better at it and it will be less uncomfortable. Make no mistake, it will never be easy, but it will hurt less.

Reason # 4: I Have Arthritis in My Knees/Hips/Back and Can't Move Well

This one's easy: water-walk or swim. The pool is the best place for people with arthritis. Find a water aerobics class and you'll have plenty of company and a great motivator. Self-conscious about getting into a bathing suit? Who isn't? Here's the thing about the pool: Once you get into the water you are essentially covered from the water line down. The walk from the change room to the pool is by far the scariest part, but you will be so proud of yourself after you do it just once. I'm not going to tell you that no one cares what you look like in a bathing suit, but the truth is that they really don't. The biggest thing to remember is this: You never know what kind of superhero you are until you put yourself up to a challenge. Just do it once and see what happens.

Reason #5: I Have No Time to Exercise

Who does? Most of us see exercise as a time-intensive activity we have to fit into our already taxing days. We see going to the gym as a two-hour event, and an exercise class is out of the question.

The key is to fit activity and exercise into your day. Find ways to fit exercise into the tasks you are already doing. Here are some classic ways to add exercise into your regular day:

1. When you take the kids to hockey practice, walk up and down the stairs at the rink. Is it soccer practice? Walk around the soccer pitch. Newsflash: Your kid won't care if you don't watch the entire practice.
2. Take twenty minutes over your lunch hour to go for a walk.
3. Before you leave work for the day, go outside and go for a thirty-minute walk. Then get in your car and drive home. If you are home thirty minutes later from work the world will not end.
4. Get up twenty minutes earlier in the morning and walk on your treadmill in your pajamas. You don't need to change, and you can even pour yourself a coffee and drink it while you walk.
5. Ever thought of riding your bike to work? How about taking public transit and getting off a few stops early and walking the rest of the way? If this is even a remote option, see if you can make it happen.

Reason #6: I'm Too Tired to Exercise

I know you're tired, but just do twenty minutes of exercise a day—your life is worth twenty minutes. If you don't have twenty minutes, you need to restructure your life to make that happen. Tell yourself that it's just twenty minutes and then see how tired you are after the twenty minutes are up.

If your life is really that crazy that you don't have twenty minutes, you need a piece of exercise equipment in your home. Chances are good that you probably have two cars, two television sets, a computer, and a cellphone. In other words, you have a variety of equipment geared toward making your life more convenient. You need one piece of equipment in your life geared toward making your life healthier.

Reason #7: I Am Embarrassed to Go to a Gym or a Pool

Who said you had to go to a gym or a pool? Get a pair of running shoes and go for a walk outside or in a mall. Start with ten minutes twice a day and build from there. If you can't walk, there are a number of exercise programs that are chair based and involve sitting exercises. You will find that after a few months of being active your confidence will skyrocket and you might find yourself in a pool or at a gym before you know it.

Reason #8: I Don't Even Know Where to Start

Start with just twenty minutes a day. I find walking to be the easiest thing to do because we all know how to do it. Increase your walking time by five minutes every two weeks until you are up to forty-five to sixty minutes a day.

Another thing to consider is a personal trainer. I'm a fan of personal trainers. I think most people erroneously think that personal trainers are both expensive and only for fit people. Wrong. A session with a personal trainer is the same price as a family dinner out at a restaurant. The trainer can give you a set of home exercises to do on your own time and tailor it to suit your needs. Further, you may find you only need a couple of sessions with the trainer, or you may find that the expense is worth it and find something else that can be budgeted out of your life to accommodate the change.

Let's go back to Elaine. Elaine falls into the category of someone who both does not like to exercise and who feels exhausted at the end of the day. Elaine loves to read books, and she also enjoys being read to—reading is Elaine's passion. I suggest she try a book on tape. This will allow her to still have her book, but at the same time she can be out for a walk. I put Elaine on my twenty-minute plan. Every night at 7 P.M. she is to go for a walk for twenty minutes along with her book on tape. After two weeks, I ask Elaine to increase her twenty minutes to twenty-five minutes and return to see me in a month.

I'm very clear with Elaine about our goals here: She will not lose any weight in this month. Let's be frank—Elaine has not made any changes in her food choices and she is going to walk an extra 140 minutes a week. If we do the math, walking for 140 minutes will allow her to burn approximately 900 calories for the week (Elaine weighs 190 pounds). There are 4000 calories in a pound, so at best she'll lose a pound this month.

The issue with Elaine goes beyond weight loss. Elaine will dramatically reduce her risk of heart attack and stroke just by beginning to exercise, but she needs to know that exercise will not result in a dramatic change to the number on the scale. When she steps on the scale in a month she cannot get discouraged because it has not moved, which is a reaction I see time and time again. People have unrealistic expectations about what exercise can do for them, and when they see the discrepancy between the treadmill and the scale they decide that it is just not worth it.

Here's the real message: You can't measure the benefits the treadmill will bring. Don't rely on the scale to tell you what you are getting from regular exercise. As you've seen from the science, the change you *will* see doesn't show up on the scale, but it may result in a different cardiovascular future. We don't have a machine to measure that benefit as yet, but give us time ... I'm sure we'll figure something out.

9

Keeping Up the Change

Anyone will tell you that making a change is one thing, but keeping it is quite another. Much of my practice is spent focusing on helping people continue to make healthy life choices and changes. Much of what I do every day is try to cement patterns of new behaviour so that they stick. This is, in fact, a bigger challenge than deciding to make a healthy life change in the first place. There are two key concepts that are essential to making a long-term, consistent life change. The first concept is what I call the "here and now." This concept aims to give you strategies for how to be happy in the moment. Your weight-loss goals are ultimately a lifelong endeavour, and we can all get impatient. The key is to learn how to be satisfied with little everyday changes. The second concept, "the new normal," will teach you how to adjust to the changes you have made and how to incorporate them into your everyday life in such a way that they are, indeed, the new normal. Let's get started.

Being Happy with the Here and Now

If you recall, I mentioned earlier how diets, by their very nature, have a beginning, middle, and an end. Implied in this is that you can restrict your calories and increase your exercise for a finite period of time and then "be done with it" and return to your previous way of life as a thinner you. Let's look at some of the ways your body's chemistry and physiology won't allow this to happen.

What we do when we diet and alter our caloric intake, regardless of our size, is to increase the body's hunger hormones in response. Ghrelin is one of the strongest hunger hormones in the body. Like many hormones, ghrelin operates based on a daily cycle. Ghrelin levels peak before meal times and are suppressed by food ingestion. They also steadily begin to rise after about 8 P.M., which could be a possible explanation of nighttime hunger in many people.[63]

Studies have shown that ghrelin levels actually rise during weight loss. One trial took fifteen healthy men without any weight issues and placed them on a calorie-restricted diet. Ghrelin levels were measured in these men frequently during the day both before caloric restriction and after. After less than a week of caloric restriction, the ghrelin levels in these men had risen by more than 20 percent. Their ghrelin levels still obeyed the peaks and valleys found in healthy subjects, but the overall levels of ghrelin were significantly higher. These men, now on a calorie-restricted diet, were hormonally on high alert against starvation.[64] Other studies have shown that dramatic changes occur in certain hormone levels in response to weight loss. These hormone levels, particularly ones that govern hunger and satiety and our response to food, remain altered for considerable periods of time after weight loss, which may account for why so many people regain weight after a significant loss.[65]

There is reassurance here in that there is a point when the brain resets some of its biochemical hardwiring, but it takes time. This is why setting goals can sometimes be more counterproductive than we initially thought. This isn't meant to discourage you from trying to lose weight, but to reassure you that this process should not have a beginning, a middle, and an end. Instead, weight loss should have only a beginning, or rather, a place to begin over and over again.

Unfortunately, human beings don't think that way. We focus instead on finite things. Movies, television shows, parties, and even our relationships have a beginning, a middle, and an end. We are structured to exist in these three phases. Even our lives have a beginning, a middle, and an end. So, how do we change a mindset that is ingrained in everything we do? The answer is simple: We focus on the first two phases—the beginning and the middle. Let's be honest: The end of this healthy journey is the end, and that's not really helpful. Most people think of the end of a diet as the place where they will have achieved their goals. That is in part true, but most people will use a diet's end as their "permission" to go back to the way things once were—to return to unhealthy habits.

So let's determine right now that this lifestyle change has to work differently. This lifestyle change must *only* have a beginning and a middle—it must focus on the everyday. I call it instead a "here" and a "now." In this way, we focus on the small steps we are taking every day and the changes we are making in this moment. We don't look at long-term goals because they are too far away; we look at what we are doing *today* and make one change in this moment.

The Power of Happiness

Psychologists talk extensively about happiness. In fact, there is an entire realm of psychology devoted to happiness. Dr. Shawn Achor, a psychologist from Harvard University, is one such expert. He has suggested that we often set success as "goal posts" for our happiness. We make statements such as "When I finish university, then I'll be happy"; "When I get my kids into a good school, I'll be happy"; "When I make partner or get married to a wonderful person or buy a new house, then I will be happy." But thinking like this puts us at a disadvantage. Dr. Achor has outlined much of this disadvantaged thinking in his groundbreaking book, *The Happiness Advantage*.[66] He points out that when we put such conditions on our happiness, we have to surpass a certain benchmark of success to achieve emotional bliss. I suggest that we do this with weight loss as well. I see it all the time with my patients: "When I lose weight I'll be happy." Many people go so far as to put a numerical amount of pounds on their happiness price: "When I lose ten, twenty, or even fifty pounds I'll be happy." When did happiness begin to have such a cost?

It's true that a lack of happiness is linked with excess weight. In fact, a study published in the *New England Journal of Medicine* in 1993 showed that 40 percent of obese women also suffered from depression.[67] Further studies have shown that weight loss does in fact improve people's quality of life and their sense of well-being.[68] This should be no surprise. What is interesting is that the studies don't show when this change happens. When did people who were losing weight get happier? Was it at the start of their weight loss? Was it after a certain amount of weight loss? What amount of pounds needs to be lost to make someone happy? The answer is that we don't know. In my experience, everyone has a different set point and often it is not the number but the process that flips the happiness switch, so to speak.

I suggest that we take a lesson from Dr. Achor. Let's not set our goal posts as hurdles that we have to leap over to attain happiness. And let's change our language from "When I lose weight I will be happy" to "I am happy that I am doing something healthier in my life right now to lose weight." Dr. Achor talks about making a list of affirmations that will help us live in the present and approach things from a positive place. Weight loss and lifestyle changes, by their very nature, need positivity to flourish. I think of my own journey with weight loss. Perhaps by design, but more likely by accident, I never had a weight-loss goal. Instead I have always maintained that I will try today to be healthier than I was yesterday. That was all. I will never set happiness as a prize on the other side of the weight-loss fence.

Studies show that our ability to see stress as a challenge and to apply positivity to our situations make us 75 percent more effective in these situations.[69] Dr. Achor calls this the "happiness advantage." From a biochemical perspective, our positivity in various situations allows dopamine to flood into our brains. Dopamine is a powerful "happy hormone" that improves productivity and is also a satiety hormone, which makes you feel full.

If we take a lesson from *The Happiness Advantage* we can apply it to weight loss. We can use the concept of positivity to embrace current changes and to maximize the effect they are having in our lives. In doing so we again focus on the here and now and the everyday changes we are making.

Step 1: Gain Perspective

Many of us can lose a sense of perspective along this road to a lifestyle change. We forget why we are making the changes we are making, and we become unsure that the changes we have already made are still in place.

To help you gain some perspective, there are two things you should do:

1. Make a list of five habits you would like to change regarding your food choices.
2. Make a list of two habits you would like to change regarding your exercise.

This may seem a bit abstract to you, so let's use one of my patients as an example. I would like you to meet Fiona, a thirty-five-year-old, happily married mother of two who is also a Grade 5 teacher. She loves her job and she loves her life. She first came to see me over five years ago. She was not active and she was an emotional eater. Dinners with her extended family and summer holidays were times when she would "go off the rails." She would allow stressful situations to be the reason for her to indulge, and she was easily gaining about five pounds per year.

Fiona finds keeping a food diary to be a huge challenge, but she knows that it helps her stay on track. Over the period of the last five years she has lost fifty pounds. She is physically active at least five days a week, attending an exercise class of some kind on each of those days. She did not magically find the time to fit these classes into her busy days; instead, she started like all my patients, with twenty to thirty minutes a day after school, and somehow her life expanded to accommodate. She realizes the power her extended family has over her emotions and now goes to family dinners with a set of rules regarding what she will eat. And she starts every summer off with a set of do's and don'ts regarding diet and exercise to give her some structure.

Fiona, in short, has a whole new approach to life and a whole new relationship with food compared to five years ago. Most importantly, she's been consistent for the last five years—rest assured, this is who she is. The problem is that she does not know that. Fiona only sees where she is now and still focuses on the fact that she has fifty more pounds to lose. In her mind, when she tackles these next fifty pounds all will be well. My goal is to get her to see how far she has come and to celebrate the journey thus far. If she can do that, she can literally be happy in *this* moment and therefore be positive about what the future brings.

I ask Fiona to make a list of the five things she is most proud of thus far in terms of her lifestyle changes. Her list looks like this:

1. I exercise almost every day.
2. My "treats" are much healthier than they used to be and I have them much less frequently. Before, I was eating cookies or chips almost daily. Now, it is one to two times a week.
3. We no longer have junk food in the house.
4. We no longer drink our calories.
5. At family dinners I am no longer out of control.

Fiona looks at her list and sees how far she has come. It is her benchmark. It has nothing to do with a goal—it is where she is now and it shows her how far she has come. Furthermore, it's a futile, difficult exercise for her because she finds it really hard to sum up all she has accomplished over the last five years in just five short sentences. Exactly.

When people ask me how my life has changed since I lost weight I laugh. How my life has *not* changed is probably a much shorter list. The important thing to remember is that our lives are fluid and they do change—if we change them. We don't look back often enough at all we have accomplished and celebrate it. Instead we try to set new goal posts that are marked with "happiness conditions." As you will see in the next step, setting goals is an important step in achieving success. However, never underestimate the importance of reflecting back on your achievements and celebrating them as you continue to push yourself forward.

Step 2: Set Positive Goals

Normally we set goals for ourselves that are focused on more than just happiness. We set our goal post at a certain point, and then move it farther away every time we get close to it. For Fiona it was "When I lose fifty pounds I'll be happy." Here she is, fifty pounds lighter, and she is still not happy. She has moved the goal post of happiness so that her brain never gets to happy.

Instead, I want her to set positive goals. In fact, studies show that if we endorse positivity in the present all levels of productivity rise. This has been shown in a variety of cases in both business and social situations.[70]

Interestingly, studies also show that positivity and realistic expectations help in weight loss. A large-scale trial in Italy published in *Behaviour Research and Therapy* in 2009 showed that a positive relationship with a patient's weight-loss counsellor had the strongest correlation to weight-loss success.[71] The study further confirmed that patients were more likely to stick with a weight-loss program if they had a more realistic expectation going into the program itself.

So I ask Fiona to pick two things she would like to improve upon in the next year that are not related to the numbers on the scale.

One should be related to food, and the other should be related to activity. Her list looked like this:

1. I would like to be better at keeping a food diary.
2. I would like to try a new physical activity, perhaps a new boot camp or even join a running club.

In this we have established some new, positive changes for Fiona to work on that are not so much goal related but are more process related.

Step 3: Practise Positive Affirmation

I want Fiona to be happy in the here and now. Many of us say we are happy and positive, but most of us can't itemize how. Having to list the things that make us happy allows us to relive the things we are grateful for.

I ask Fiona to make a list of things she is grateful for from her weight-loss journey. She brings back the following:

1. My family is really supportive of this process.
2. My kids are asking for healthier food overall.
3. I have far more energy.
4. I have more structure in my life regarding food choices.
5. I eat healthier.
6. I "get it" more; I feel more in control and happier.
7. I like shopping—clothes fit me better.
8. I have more confidence.
9. I like my life more.

I ask Fiona to write down one thing every day for a month that she is grateful for relating to her lifestyle change. This allows her to reflect upon one new thing every day.

Fiona is a perfect example of someone who, from the outside, has made amazing changes in her life but she can't see the forest for the trees. She initially felt disenchanted with the process because she felt that she was not making any progress. By allowing her to look at where she has come from, to be in a positive place now, and to look to the future from that place of positivity she can celebrate her accomplishments and move forward with a positive outlook. According to the psychology of happiness, she is far more likely to be productive and even more likely to enjoy the process overall. In summary, remember to do the following:

- Live in the here and now—focus on your daily changes and how far you've come.
- Have a sense of perspective along the way.
- Set positive goals.
- Reaffirm positivity every day.

If we try these steps while going through this process we will find that we are not only more productive in our commitment to health, but we also no longer see it as the things we left behind.

Often within this process we balance between what we have and don't have, where we are and where we have yet to get to. The point of being in the here and now is to shift our thinking from these two polarizing views. Instead, we focus on today—how far we have come and what we have now. We no longer come to this process from a place where all we see are the things we can't do, the foods we can't eat, and the fun times we left behind. Instead, we focus on the opportunities around us, the health we have *now,* and the important milestones we've accomplished thus far.

The New Normal

Have you ever heard of the phenomenon called phantom limb syndrome? It occurs when a patient loses a limb, most commonly his or her leg, to an amputation and the brain continues to think that the limb is still there.[72] Our brains are pretty elaborate organs that have an intricate network of systems that allow us to move our bodies through this world. The part of the brain that monitors our own sense of "space" is the somatosensory cortex, which is located in the postcentral gyrus. This part of the brain receives sensory input from our body and helps us get a sense of ourselves in space. When we lose a limb our brains need time to adjust to the change in space, so to speak. When I lost weight I went through a form of phantom limb syndrome. In my mind I was always much bigger than I was in reality. The scale said one thing but my brain somehow could not adjust to what my new physical reality was.

When applied to weight loss, phantom limb syndrome goes beyond this disconnect between what used to be and what is now. I call this "the new normal." I will maintain that "normal" is a moving target. What is a normal diet? What's a normal exercise plan? Doesn't normal move and change and shift over time? Don't we adapt to our surroundings from time to time such that there is always a new normal for us to compare to? By its very nature, change demands that we establish a new normal in everything we do.

The important thing in this process is for you to do the same. You need to adapt to the changes that this new life brings, reflecting on what is "normal" now and where you want to get to in terms of a healthier future. Like any change, however, you will find that the lessons are everywhere around you.

Last week I was at a party with some friends I had not seen in some time. A dear friend of mine asked what I had been up to and I mentioned that I was writing a book.

"Oh? What's it about?" she inquired.

"It's about how to make a lifestyle change," I answered, trying to sum up all my ideas in one sentence.

"So how's it done?" she asked.

"With great difficulty," I laughed.

Our conversation went on from there and somehow we got on the topic of exercise. I had just finished writing the chapter on exercise and mentioned that I was writing about the common reasons I hear in my practice for people not being able to exercise. I should say that my friend is one of the most driven, high-achieving women I know. She really is amazing, and I am not just saying that because she will no doubt read this book. She owns her own business, is a mother of two, and has a sense of style most women would envy. In short, she is a rock star.

But something happened over the course of our discussion on why people don't exercise. Our conversation went from a friendly, loving exchange to her being overly defensive. I felt terrible and went away from our interaction feeling as though I had put my foot in my mouth. Why had I brought my work up in a social setting? Why had I felt the need to share this message at this party? Furthermore, why had my dear friend taken my conversation the wrong way? Didn't she know that I was just discussing the book I was writing, like I would tell any anecdote at a party? Why was this discussion so personal?

And then it became clear. This lifestyle change—the idea of eating better and exercising more—is intensely personal. *Everyone* has an opinion about this, not just my friend, and his or her opinion is often laced with a deep emotional and personal attachment. My friend was defensive about my discussion because, for whatever reason, her life reflected something I had discussed.

I have seen this many times before in my travels. I will be on a plane and someone will ask me what I do. When I tell him or her that I am a doctor, the inevitable question arises: "Oh, what kind of doctor?"

"I'm a specialist in internal medicine and obesity."

"Obesity?" they ask. "So you try and help people lose weight?"

"Yes, I do," I answer.

"Oh." There is a silence. If they are eating one of the snacks on the plane, they look down to make sure their food choice is appropriate. Sometimes they will ask me about their own behaviours, other times they'll ask about a friend or family member who is overweight or obese. Sometimes they will share with me an observation or an opinion regarding the state of health in this country.

Ultimately, I have realized how personal diet and exercise are. Everyone—and I mean everyone—has some sort of dieting experience. They have either been on a diet or are living with someone who has. They undoubtedly have a parent or co-worker or spouse who has in some way tried to change their eating habits. As such, they inevitably have a bias of some kind toward this process.

What my friend taught me in that moment was that this process is about an individual's *normal*. Everyone has a sense of reality that, regardless of its benefits or drawbacks, works for them in some way. When I discussed the reasons why people don't exercise my friend saw herself. She automatically jumped to the assumption that I do not understand her life, its complexities, and where she is coming from. Her normal was different from mine. Moreover, there was no room in her normal for any adjustments at that time. For me to suggest such a thing was an affront to her way of life, and therefore I had inadvertently made a personal attack.

As you are reading this book I am sure you will find certain parts that do to you what my conversation did to my friend at the party. There are certain points where you will undoubtedly think, "Who does she think she is?" or "Easier said than done." Make no mistake, I hear you.

I understand that this is a very personal process, and regardless of how hard you try, your ego will take a hit along the way. This process of change is *not* easy and it is very personal. It forces you to look at your life and see what is wrong with it. How much of a kick in the face is that?

Try instead to focus on the idea of "normal" as a moving target. There is no judgment here. I know your life is not where you want it to be. If it were, you would not be reading this book. I know you want to change something about the way you look at food and exercise and health. But here's the problem when we make it too personal: We lose sight of what work needs to be done.

Here's an exercise for you: Think about what part of what I have said so far in this book has upset you. (Maybe you've stopped reading already and you aren't able to participate in my little activity, but I hope not!) But if you *are* still reading this book, what part made you a bit angry? *That very part is likely most reflective of something in your own life that you want to change.*

When I was in residency I had a mentor, Dr. Harvey Rabin, who really made me a better doctor. To this day, almost thirteen years later, I can still hear his voice in my head. He taught me that if I am ever uncomfortable with a patient interaction it is likely that there is something in my own personal life that needs adjusting. This was one of his greatest teachings to me, and it involved a very difficult interaction with a patient. I was doing a rotation in infectious diseases at the time and Dr. Rabin was my preceptor. We were asked to consult on a patient who was morbidly obese. He was forty-two years old, a type 2 diabetic, and had been admitted to hospital with a heart attack but had developed a diabetic foot infection during his stay. Recall at the time that I was easily 150 pounds overweight. Now, I should say that I may not be the smartest doctor or the best diagnostician, but I'm pretty good at bedside manner. In residency, that was my strong point. I loved being at the bedside with patients and their families—*that* was my thing. Somehow, though, with this patient it was different. Every time I went in the room I felt like I could not wait to get out of there. I was unusually brief with my interactions.

As was usual protocol I went to see the patient first. I was uncharacteristically brief when taking a history and doing a physical exam. This man lay there in bed, barely able to move because his size was prohibitive. Every nurse who was involved in his care had a comment of some kind on his size. Every note in the chart made it glaringly obvious that he was *morbidly obese* and difficult to examine. I could not help but notice the cans of pop and packets of candy on his bedside table and had a knee-jerk reaction about their appropriateness. I was ashamed instantly at my inability to empathize.

I gathered my findings as best I could, but I was not focused on the case at all. I went to present my findings to Dr. Rabin and it was a disaster. This was a simple consult on a diabetic foot infection and I was all over the place.

Dr. Rabin stopped me midway and asked, "Ali, what's wrong with you?"

"I'm just tired." Sure, I was tired—it was residency and I had not slept in four years. But it was more than that. I started to cry. Never mind that I was crying, I was crying in front of one of my favourite teachers and mentors. This was an all-time low.

But he handed me a tissue and did the one thing the very best mentors always do: He gave me advice that to this day remains true in life and in medicine.

"Ali," he said with sincerity, "when something bothers you with a patient, ask yourself why. What about this interaction pushed the wrong buttons? Is it just the sadness of the case? Or is it something about *your* life that speaks to you?"

I'd like to say that I went home that day and instantly made a commitment to a healthier life, but I'd be lying. It took a few years for me to begin my path to health. The lesson of that day was different: When something makes you angry or sad or triggers a pretty basic impulse of emotion it is usually because it has struck a nerve about your own life. And the same thing holds true about the advice in this book.

So here is one more piece of advice: Check yourself. Check what has spoken to you in such a personal way to elicit that kind of response—the same one my friend had at the party or the same one I had at that patient's bedside. That is the place to start. There is something there that speaks to you and is beckoning for change. Now go answer the call.

Anytime we challenge the normal we trigger that response. The key is to understand that "normal" is our own perception of what is normal. In today's society we've done so much to skew what normal really is: Kids today think it's normal to have a pop machine in school; a frappuccino is viewed as a perfectly acceptable breakfast coffee; and anyone who exercises every day is anything but normal. When we challenge the normal we threaten our own life balance—we feel a leg where there is none.

The key here is to establish a new normal. We teach amputees to slowly retrain their brains toward the loss of a limb. I learned from Dr. Rabin that I was not angry with my obese diabetic patient, I was angry at myself. My friend got defensive because she would like to have more time to exercise in her otherwise crazy life. Normal is a moving target. Many of us wake up years into a life and wonder, "How did I get here?"

Here's the thing: Breathe. Take one step at a time and establish a new normal. Set small goals for yourself and then get to them. Rejoice in the process that is helping you reset what is normal.

Lewis is thirty-four years old. His life is an example of "normal as a moving target." He has struggled through a variety of life challenges, each of which resets what he perceives as normal. Lewis was a fit, healthy twenty-three-year-old man when he was diagnosed with leukemia. He had been an avid runner and was training for his first marathon when he noticed that he was far more fatigued and short of breath than he should have been. A visit to his family doctor showed that his blood counts were dangerously abnormal and he was immediately admitted to the hospital. After a series of bone marrow tests, Lewis was diagnosed with acute myeloid leukemia. He underwent several rounds of chemotherapy and then a bone marrow transplant. There were complications along the way, including two ICU admissions for severe sepsis when Lewis's doctors thought he might die. He suffered severe muscle wasting and a fractured hip as a result of the steroids. The entire process took eighteen months until he was finally given the "all clear."

Lewis is a soft-spoken man whose kindness almost fills the room he sits in. He speaks matter-of-factly about how, when he finished all of his chemotherapy, his body had changed dramatically:

> I looked nothing like the marathoner that went into the hospital. At first, through the chemo and the stem cell transplant, I had lost so much weight and so much muscle mass that I was emaciated. Then once the steroids came on board I could not gain weight fast enough. People kept bringing me milkshakes to the hospital. I had mouth sores and they were the only things I could drink for a while. I must have had five or six per day. I reasoned that they would help me put on weight; I had cancer, after all. I also reasoned that as long as I was gaining weight I wasn't sick. It was this bizarre series of rationalizations. I could eat whatever I wanted because I was sick, and if I gained weight I wasn't sick. I had come a long way from the guy who was the nutrition freak who ran eight miles a day.

Lewis is now more than a decade beyond his diagnosis. He receives annual checkups and continues to be in remission. He is now a lawyer and engaged to a wonderful woman. His life looks nothing like it did on the day of his diagnosis, nor does it bear any resemblance to the one he had on the day he was discharged from hospital. Lewis is 5-foot-10 and weighs 230 pounds. He leads a pretty sedentary life.

"I'm a sugar addict. I always was, but before, when I was running, I could get away with it. Then I had the chemo and, well, you know how that goes. Now I eat way too many sweets and it just all fell apart. Now, sure, I'm healthy, but I don't know where to begin."

Yes, there are a host of reasons why Lewis's physical condition changed as a result of his cancer. As a physician I view this reconditioning as unfortunate, but I am grateful that Lewis is alive and able to face his daily challenges healthy and happy. Lewis agrees.

He does not mourn the loss of his marathon self; instead, he realizes that normal is a moving target.

As human beings we are constantly faced with challenges that force us to adapt and move on. The key with a healthy new lifestyle is to use those adaptive techniques in your new way of life. I have seen it countless times before. Lewis teaches us that people are incredibly resilient and adaptive. Although change is shocking and unsettling, we adjust to it in a frighteningly adaptive way. We just need to have faith in the process and in our abilities and trust that our normal will be re-established. Let's leave this chapter with words from Lewis:

> Sure it would be great to be *that guy* again. But I'm not. I've seen too much and experienced too much. That guy had it easy. I was in my early twenties, I was fit, and all I had to worry about was what my last run time was. When I first got diagnosed with leukemia I was pissed off. I did the usual "why me?" But you adapt. I was in hospital for almost a year. The place was like my home. You adapt. Now I'm, like, sixty pounds overweight. You adapt. The difference now is that I don't want *this* to be the way it's going to be. If I have to adapt again, I want to adapt to something healthier. So I know I can handle this. Every time I feel sorry for myself that I'm no longer the runner who was really fit I'm going to remember how strong I really am. I survived leukemia. I can survive obesity. This does not have to be the way it is forever. Sure, maybe this weight served a purpose up until now. But it's not working for me anymore and I need to find a new healthier state. Make no mistake, Dr. Zentner, I don't feel sorry for myself. I also don't feel like it's my fault that I gained all this weight. It doesn't matter anymore who or what is responsible. Knowing that won't really help me get healthy. I just have to take it upon myself to get there. I have to believe that I *can* find a totally

different healthy place to be that looks nothing like what I perceived health to be before. Before, health was either being a marathon runner or not having cancer. I have to find a new healthy place to be and make that my own. Yeah, I know I can get there.

Amen, Lewis. Amen.

10

How to Keep a Food Diary

As you have likely already figured out, I am a big fan of keeping a food diary. There is an overwhelming amount of scientific evidence that shows that this is a useful weight-loss tool. A study published in the *American Journal of Preventative Medicine* is one such large-scale trial. In this study, 1685 overweight or obese adults were asked to keep food diaries as part of a weight-loss program. The patients who kept a food diary lost twice as much weight as those who did not at the end of six months.[73] Critically speaking, one could argue that the more "motivated" patients were more likely to keep a food diary and therefore were more likely to lose a greater amount of weight. That being said, motivation is not just born, it is also made.

Think about this: When you engage in any lifestyle change there are often a variety of negatives. As I mentioned in the chapter on exercise, we focus too much on what we can't do, where we can't eat, and what we are missing out on. A food diary should put the focus on what you are doing now and where the changes need to be made.

Here are some basic rules to follow when you keep a food diary:

1. **Keep it honest.** Your food diary is for your eyes only. This is about what you are doing and what you are eating. If you are going to get "creative" with your food recording, it is not going to be a reflection of what you are truly eating.
2. **Don't beat yourself up.** This has to be a positive process. It's not grade school and it's not a test—you will not be judged or graded on the quality of your recording nor on the food you record.
3. **We learn by making mistakes.** When you go through your diary entries at the end of the day, be kind. Instead of asking yourself "Why did I eat that?" which implies a scolding is needed, ask "What can I do differently next time?" A positive approach is key.

Where to Start: The Basics

When you first begin to keep a food diary, decide if you are going to do it online or with a plain old pen and paper. I'm often asked which is better, but it really does not matter. In fact, a study published in 2007 asked this exact question. The study randomized two groups of obese and overweight people to one of two forms of food diary recording. One group was given a PDA (personal digital assistant) and instructed to use an online form of a food diary. The other group was given pen and paper and asked to write down everything they ate. At the end of six months the results from each group were revealed and compared, and it turns out that both groups did about the same in terms of weight loss *and* both groups felt satisfied with their form of food diary recording.[74] The take-home message here is that it does not matter how you record your food diary, only that you do record it. The ideal format for you is the one you are most likely to use.

If you are going to go the pen-and-paper route, then get a designated notebook or a small notepad—you may want something that can travel with you or alternatively something that can be left in a central place in your home. Ideally you want something that you can use throughout the day. I personally like my food diary to be stylish. I figure it's a pretty important book, so I go for classic black moleskin. In my mind there is something to the idea that I've "treated" myself to a lovely little notebook.

Many people tell me that they find it a challenge to keep track of their food as they eat during the day. Remember, this is an exercise that you just have to do for a week at a time. When you break down the task into a seven-day period it is not quite so onerous. There are then several ways to start keeping a food diary.

Step 1: The Basics

For seven days write down everything you eat. Try and do it right after a meal while it is still fresh in your mind. Remember that studies show people engaging in this process *under-record* what they are eating by at least 10 percent, so be honest.

Step 2: Be Specific

The most effective food diaries are the ones that are very specific regarding the amounts of food eaten. So try and be specific in terms of how much you have eaten. For example, "Two pieces of whole-wheat toast with 2 tbsp of peanut butter" is much more helpful than "Toast with peanut butter." This only needs to be done for a day or two. I've given you an example of a specific food diary on the following page.

Specific Food Diary

Sunday	Monday	Tuesday	Wednesday	Thursday	Friday	Saturday
2 eggs 2 pieces of turkey bacon 1 tomato, sliced 1/2 cup fruit salad 2 pieces of toast with 2 tbsp of peanut butter	1/2 cup fruit salad 2 pieces of toast with 2 tbsp of peanut butter	1/2 cup fruit salad 2 pieces of toast with 2 tbsp of peanut butter	1/2 cup fruit salad 2 pieces of toast with 2 tbsp of peanut butter	1/2 cup fruit salad 2 pieces of toast with 2 tbsp of peanut butter	1/2 cup fruit salad 2 pieces of toast with 2 tbsp of peanut butter	1/2 cup fruit salad 2 pieces of toast with 2 tbsp of peanut butter
2 cups canned tomato soup 2 pieces of whole-wheat bread 3 slices of cheddar cheese 2 tbsp butter	2 cups meat chili 2 slices of garlic toast	Turkey sandwich (2 pieces of whole-wheat bread with mustard, 4 ounces sliced turkey, lettuce, tomato) 1 small yogurt Apple Granola bar	Turkey sandwich (2 pieces of whole-wheat bread with mustard, 4 ounces sliced turkey, lettuce, tomato) 1 small yogurt Apple Granola bar	Turkey sandwich (2 pieces of whole-wheat bread with mustard, 4 ounces sliced turkey, lettuce, tomato 1 small yogurt Apple Granola bar	6-inch ham sub 1 small chicken noodle soup 1 chocolate chip cookie	Cheeseburger Small fries Diet pop (restaurant)
1.5 cups pasta 1 cup meat sauce 2 cups romaine lettuce with 3 tbsp Caesar dressing	6 ounces chicken breast 2 cups of veggies 2 tbsp olive oil	6 ounces roasted pork chop 1 cup of sweet potatoes Salad with 2 tbsp of dressing	6-ounce steak Baked potato Caesar salad (restaurant)	Stir-fry (6 ounces shrimp, 2 cups of veggies, 2 tbsp olive oil, 2 tsp of soy sauce, 1 tsp of honey, ginger) 1 cup of rice	Fettuccine Alfredo 1 piece of cheesecake 2 glasses of wine (restaurant)	2 cups meat chili 2 slices of garlic toast Salad with 2 tbsp of low-fat dressing

Step 3: Reflection

At the end of every day look at what you have eaten. Highlight the choices that you made that could have been healthier and the areas that you have issues with. Reflect upon where you want to make changes. Remember, *this is not a time to beat yourself up*. As human beings we learn by our mistakes. So settle down, lose the judgment, and start looking at your own behaviour and seeing where you can improve upon it.

If we take the example on the next page, you can see areas that I've highlighted that could be improved upon.

Step 4: Develop a Sense of Food Economy

I highly recommend that you take your food diary one step further and see how many calories you are eating at each interval. By their nature, food diaries give us a sense of food economy, meaning a sense of how much we are eating and where our calories are being spent. But to take that one step further, count your calories for a given day or days. You can see how many calories are in the foods you eat by reading labels or going online and searching for their calorie totals. This involves a bit more work, but it does not need to be done every day—you just need to do it for a week. What you then see is where you are *spending* most of your calories and where you can cut back. Going back to my original food diary, you can see the calorie amounts shown on pages 134 and 135.

Can you spot the problem areas? In this food diary it is rather obvious what the problem is: portion sizes and too many meals out. But you can also see how the food diary is a way for us to diagnose our own eating patterns.

Highlighted Food Diary

Sunday	Monday	Tuesday	Wednesday	Thursday	Friday	Saturday
2 eggs 2 pieces of turkey bacon 1 tomato, sliced 1/2 cup fruit salad 2 pieces of toast with 2 tbsp of peanut butter	1/2 cup fruit salad 2 pieces of toast with 2 tbsp of peanut butter	1/2 cup fruit salad 2 pieces of toast with 2 tbsp of peanut butter	1/2 cup fruit salad 2 pieces of toast with 2 tbsp of peanut butter	1/2 cup fruit salad 2 pieces of toast with 2 tbsp of peanut butter	1/2 cup fruit salad 2 pieces of toast with 2 tbsp of peanut butter	1/2 cup fruit salad 2 pieces of toast with 2 tbsp of peanut butter
2 cups canned tomato soup 2 pieces of whole-wheat bread 3 slices of cheddar cheese 2 tbsp butter	2 cups meat chili 2 slices of garlic toast	Turkey sandwich (2 pieces of whole-wheat bread with mustard, 4 ounces sliced turkey, lettuce, tomato) 1 small yogurt Apple Granola bar	Turkey sandwich (2 pieces of whole-wheat bread with mustard, 4 ounces sliced turkey, lettuce, tomato 1 small yogurt Apple Granola bar	Turkey sandwich (2 pieces of whole-wheat bread with mustard, 4 ounces sliced turkey, lettuce, tomato 1 small yogurt Apple Granola bar	6-inch ham sub 1 small chicken noodle soup 1 chocolate chip cookie	Cheeseburger Small fries Diet pop (restaurant)
1.5 cups pasta 1 cup meat sauce 2 cups romaine lettuce with 3 tbsp Caesar dressing	6 ounces chicken breast 2 cups of veggies 2 tbsp olive oil	6 ounces roasted pork chop 1 cup of sweet potatoes Salad with 2 tbsp of dressing	6-ounce steak Baked potato Caesar salad (restaurant)	Stir-fry (6 ounces shrimp, 2 cups of veggies, 2 tbsp olive oil, 2 tsp of soy sauce, 1 tsp of honey, ginger) 1 cup of rice	Fettuccine Alfredo 1 piece of cheesecake 2 glasses of wine (restaurant)	2 cups meat chili 2 slices of garlic toast Salad with 2 tbsp of low-fat dressing

"Calorie Counted" Food Diary

Sunday (2320 calories)	Monday (1540 calories)	Tuesday (1440 calories)	Wednesday (2040 calories)	Thursday (1640 calories)	Friday (2290 calories)	Saturday (1940 calories)
2 eggs 2 pieces of turkey bacon 1 tomato, sliced 1/2 cup fruit salad 2 pieces of toast with 2 tbsp of peanut butter (670 calories)	1/2 cup fruit salad 2 pieces of toast with 2 tbsp of peanut butter (440 calories)	1/2 cup fruit salad 2 pieces of toast with 2 tbsp of peanut butter (440 calories)	1/2 cup fruit salad 2 pieces of toast with 2 tbsp of peanut butter (440 calories)	1/2 cup fruit salad 2 pieces of toast with 2 tbsp of peanut butter (440 calories)	1/2 cup fruit salad 2 pieces of toast with 2 tbsp of peanut butter (440 calories)	1/2 cup fruit salad 2 pieces of toast with 2 tbsp of peanut butter (440 calories)
2 cups canned tomato soup 2 pieces of whole-wheat bread 3 slices of cheddar cheese 2 tbsp butter (880 calories)	2 cups meat chili 2 slices of garlic toast (700 calories)	Turkey sandwich (2 pieces of whole-wheat bread with mustard, 4 ounces sliced turkey, lettuce, tomato) 1 small yogurt Apple Granola bar (600 calories)	Turkey sandwich (2 pieces of whole-wheat bread with mustard, 4 ounces sliced turkey, lettuce, tomato) 1 small yogurt Apple Granola bar (600 calories)	Turkey sandwich (2 pieces of whole-wheat bread with mustard, 4 ounces sliced turkey, lettuce, tomato) 1 small yogurt Apple Granola bar (600 calories)	6-inch ham sub 1 small chicken noodle soup 1 chocolate chip cookie (550 calories)	Cheeseburger Small fries Diet pop (restaurant) (750 calories)

Sunday (2320 calories)	**Monday (1540 calories)**	**Tuesday (1440 calories)**	**Wednesday (2040 calories)**	**Thursday (1640 calories)**	**Friday (2290 calories)**	**Saturday (1940 calories)**
1.5 cups pasta 1 cup meat sauce 2 cups romaine lettuce with 3 tbsp Caesar dressing (770 calories)	6 ounces chicken breast 2 cups of veggies 2 tbsp olive oil (400 calories)	6 ounces roasted pork chop 1 cup of sweet potatoes Salad with 2 tbsp of dressing (400 calories)	6-ounce steak Baked potato Caesar salad (restaurant) (1000 calories)	Stir-fry (6 ounces shrimp, 2 cups of veggies, 2 tbsp olive oil, 2 tsp of soy sauce, 1 tsp of honey, ginger) 1 cup of rice (600 calories)	Fettuccine Alfredo 1 piece of cheesecake 2 glasses of wine (restaurant) (1300 calories)	2 cups meat chili 2 slices of garlic toast Salad with 2 tbsp of low-fat dressing (750 calories)

A Digital Age

If you are not a fan of the pen-and-paper route, the world is your oyster. There are a variety of online food diary programs available at a minimal cost to the user. Some have a ten-day free-trial period so you can pick the one that you want. Furthermore, I'm assuming that most of you reading this have a smart phone. There are a variety of apps available that involve calorie counting and food diaries. Try one or two out and see how you do. Here are some of my favourite online food diary programs:

www.fitday.com
www.calorieking.com
www.myfooddiary.com

Learning Over Performance

The key to keeping a food diary is *not* to judge how well you performed in the process. Most people have been "messed up" in the past by keeping a food diary. Think of it this time as an entirely new process. Here are some common misconceptions and barriers to keeping a food diary:

If I Have to Write It Down I Won't Eat It

This may be true for some, but that's not the point of a food diary. I want you to see a food diary as a blueprint for change—it should reflect where you are right now and act as a proposal or a guide for where you need to make some healthy changes. A food diary is not a police officer that acts as a hindrance, preventing you from eating certain things. If you see it like that it will either encourage you to be dishonest with yourself regarding what you really did eat or it will encourage you to chastise yourself about your food choices.

I Forgot What I Ate Yesterday and Had to Sit Down at Night and Recall the Day in Reverse

This is a really common event. We all have busy lives that revolve around certain habits and rituals. Adding a new ritual into the mix can be a task, for sure. It often gets missed or overlooked. If this is the case for you, keep your food diary with you at all times just for a few days so that it becomes a visual cue for you to keep track of and record your food as you eat.

I Suck at Keeping a Food Diary

We all do. Recording our behaviour is not something we as human beings do. We are very good at being in the moment—at engaging in the behaviour. Observing our own behaviour is not our strong point. I remember in medical school being told to check my own pulse before checking the patient's in any situation. This seemed so odd to me. Why would I care about my pulse? I was not the one who was sick. The point of the exercise was for me to check my own anxiety or emotions before I engaged in a clinical encounter with someone else. As with a food diary, it's not about how well you do keeping track of your eating, it's about what you learn. Forget how good or bad you are at keeping the diary and instead see what you learn by doing it. You may only learn that you are bad at keeping a food diary. But more likely you will learn where some of your "problem areas" are regarding food. Regardless, when you focus on the process of keeping the diary and not on the result of "how well you do," you have a much better chance of having a positive learning experience.

I Don't Like Keeping a Food Diary

This is probably true for most of you, but when you think about all the things you do in a day that you don't enjoy and yet do anyway, I'm sure you can do this, too. There is so much about change that is not enjoyable, just like there is so much about body maintenance that is not enjoyable. For instance, I hate brushing my teeth—I find it onerous and really boring. But I do it. Twice a day, sometimes more. It sounds patronizing, perhaps, but does everything always have to be enjoyable to be worth doing? Can't we sometimes just do things that are less than enjoyable but that in the long term become something that we benefit from? This lifestyle change is something you will ultimately enjoy. A food diary is a step that you may not, but keep your eyes on the prize. Focus on the end result here: a healthier future and all that it implies rather than the lack of enjoyment from a daily process that, at most, takes five to ten minutes of your day.

Keeping a Food Diary Makes Me Obsess About Food

This is a common response. Many patients I see talk about how they are disenchanted with the whole process of examining their behaviour around food as it worries them that it will become an obsession. When it comes to weight loss and being overweight or obese you may have an obsession with food to begin with. I would argue that many of my obese patients already think about food frequently throughout the day. I myself love food, and I think about it often. I think about dinner at breakfast time. I think about my upcoming birthday cake and what it will look and taste like. Food is a part of who we are as a culture, and many of us do think about it pretty often throughout the day. Food diaries will not stop you from obsessing about food, but you likely do that already. The key here is that you will use your powers for good and not evil—you will think about food, but then use those thoughts to change patterns of behaviour for the better.

There you have it—the bare bones of keeping a food diary. As you can see, it really is not such a daunting process.

11

Meal Makeovers and Special Situations

Most of us know what we should be eating, but I worry that sometimes health gets lost in the translation. For example, my husband thinks that chocolate milk is healthy. He is a runner and someone once told him that the best recovery drink after a marathon is chocolate milk. From this, he somehow got it into his head that chocolate milk is healthy. Sure, the milk part of chocolate milk is most definitely healthy. However, if you add sugar and corn syrup to any healthy drink you water down the healthy benefits. I share this story not to prevent my husband from ever buying chocolate milk again (although that's not a bad idea), but to highlight for you how often what we think is healthy is really not.

So far, we've talked about different ways people can change their eating patterns, mostly by making over their meals. In this chapter, I'll give you some specific healthy meal makeover suggestions for places to start that will allow you, in your own time, to redecorate what you are eating. Furthermore, meal makeovers can happen both at home and in a restaurant; you can make healthier choices regardless of whether you eat out or stay in. So let's begin with the everyday meals that you have in your own home.

Breakfast

Breakfast really is the most important meal of the day. Recall from my little physiology lesson that our bodies are very sensitive to periods of famine and not so sensitive to periods of feast; we have evolved to be highly efficient at storing energy in the form of fat. Think about what this means if you don't eat breakfast.

There are typically three barriers I hear from my patients preventing them from eating breakfast:

1. I'm not hungry when I wake up in the morning.
2. I have no time to eat breakfast.
3. I don't like breakfast foods.

Let's address each of these with a lesson from Jamie.

I'm Not Hungry When I Wake Up

Jamie is thirty years old and she does not eat breakfast. Her dinnertime is around 7 P.M. and she'll snack sometimes in the evenings. She usually has her last bite of food at around 9 or 9:30 P.M. She gets up for work at seven o'clock in the morning and has a coffee. Jamie never eats breakfast and rarely has lunch. Her first meal is around 3 P.M., and by then she is starving.

Jamie's brain thinks she is starving, and she continues to perpetuate the myth. Further, she consumes her greatest amount of calories during her least active moments. Jamie needs to start eating breakfast. This is going to be a big change for her, and she'll likely resent me a bit since by introducing breakfast she will undoubtedly be hungry by about 10 A.M. The issue here is one of physiology. She's "turned on" the cycle of hunger and satiety hormones. That being said, she will also shift her calorie consumption to reflect her waking time.

Jamie is never hungry when she wakes up in the morning. Nonetheless, I encourage her to have something more than just coffee when she first wakes up. Here are some examples:

1. A piece of fruit
2. Yogurt
3. A smoothie made with fruit, milk, and even some protein powder
4. A protein bar

All of these items are quick, small, and easy. The protein shake is by far the best received by those people who aren't hungry in the morning, since most people in this category are likely to drink something in the morning without a problem. Therefore, having them drink their breakfast is not a big stretch.

I Have No Time to Eat Breakfast

No one has time in the mornings—mornings are crazy. The key here is to find fast and easy items that are effortless. Here are a few ideas:

1. **Oatmeal.** Oatmeal takes no time at all because it comes in an instant variety, where all you have to do is add boiling water. Alternatively, a healthier method is to make a large pot of traditional steel cut oats on the weekend and put it into small, individual-size containers and freeze them for the week. In the morning you can microwave the oatmeal at home and eat it while you are getting ready for work, or you can take it to work frozen and microwave it there.
2. **Protein bar.** This is an easy, somewhat nutritious option. I recommend you buy a variety of protein bars in single form and pick the flavour and brand you like best. Stick with protein bars that are less than 300 calories each and have around 20 grams of protein in each bar.

3. **Toast with peanut butter or cheese.** This option takes three minutes to make—I've timed it. And you can eat it in the car, if you must.
4. **Fruit and yogurt parfait.** This can be made the night before when you are making your lunch and eaten in the morning on the way to work.
5. **Cheese and crackers and a piece of fruit.** Fast, easy, and nutritious.

One of the easiest ways to have a quick breakfast in the morning is to make it the night before, perhaps when you are making dinner or your lunch for the next day. Then, when you wake up in the morning, your breakfast is waiting for you.

I Don't Like Breakfast Foods

Jamie asks me point-blank, "What do I eat for breakfast?" I respond with, "What do you like to eat?"

This is the first point of breakfast: Eat what you like. Personally, I hate breakfast foods. I usually eat a breakfast that looks very much like a lunch. Jamie loves turkey sandwiches. I suggest she take one for breakfast. My list of breakfasts for the non-breakfast eater includes the following:

1. **A sandwich of any kind.** Turkey, peanut butter and banana, you pick it. There is no reason why your breakfast can't look like your lunch. Make it the night before with your lunch and you have yourself a fast and easy solution.
2. **An omelet.** Yeah, it sounds crazy that this would be a fast option. You can make the omelet the night before and then microwave it in the morning. Most non-breakfast eaters love the idea of a Sunday breakfast, including omelets and such. The omelet can have two

eggs and lots of veggies, which makes it a wonderfully healthy option. Furthermore, the Harvard Egg Study found that eating one egg a day is as safe as eating one egg a week,[75] but if you are concerned about the cholesterol in eggs, switch to egg whites.

3. **Leftovers from dinner.** Who has not had pizza for breakfast at some point? I'm not suggesting pizza is the healthiest breakfast choice, but the concept is right on—eat your leftovers from dinner for breakfast. A piece of roasted chicken and some sweet potatoes is a really nutritious way to start the day.

Breakfast is always a tricky meal to make over for people who either don't eat it or for those who have been using breakfast as a time to eat pastry. When it comes to establishing a healthy first meal of the day, I suggest you stick to the following guidelines:

1. **No pastries of any kind.** Muffins are just cake in another form. Don't be fooled into thinking that just because it says "low fat" or "high fibre" a muffin is the way to go. The average muffin has almost the same amount of calories and fat as a Big Mac.
2. **Eat something.** If you aren't a breakfast eater, start small and build from there.
3. **Make your breakfast the night before or even at the start of the week.** Leave it in the fridge or freezer and you can eat it en route to work or even while you are getting ready in the morning.
4. **Eat what you like in the morning.** Don't force yourself to have cereal if you hate it. If you are trying to turn yourself on to breakfast it should consist of foods you at least find palatable.

Lunch

Now that we've tackled breakfasts, let's move on to lunches. For both lunches and dinners I want you to think of your plate like you would a room. You would never have a living room without chairs and a couch—a *living* room has to have the components for *living,* just like a bedroom needs a bed. Similarly, a meal needs nutritional components just like a room needs the components for its purpose.

Remember when we were little and we took our lunches to school? Packing a lunch was standard fare for most of us before the age of twelve. This is something we are all familiar with, but many of us have lost the concept along the way. As a rule I recommend bringing lunch with you to work or school whenever possible. It will automatically give you nutritional control over what you are eating and reinforce certain mindful eating initiatives that you have already undertaken.

When it comes to packing a lunch or even eating out at lunch the components are easy:

- It should be convenient. Most people will want their lunch to be portable, especially if they are taking it to work or school.
- It should be nutritious. Rather than telling you exactly what to eat, try incorporating the following into your lunches:

  1 serving of protein (4–6 ounces)
  1–2 servings of starch
  2–3 servings of vegetables
  1 fruit
  1 serving of dairy

Remember, serving sizes should be logical. A piece of bread or a piece of fruit is one serving. If you are looking at measurable items, either 1/2 cup or 1 cup is a measurable serving, or 4–6 ounces when it comes to protein. Here are some basic ideas that should act as building blocks for a healthier lunch:

1. **Sandwich.** Pick a protein—chicken, turkey, salmon, tuna—put it on whole-wheat bread, and add vegetables to it. Combine it with a piece of fruit and a yogurt and you are good to go. Add some extra cut-up vegetables to the mix and you have a pretty nutritious lunch.
2. **Salad.** This is a sandwich minus the bread. Pile on the vegetables; add some protein and even an ounce or two of cheese. The key here is to watch that you don't pile on the dressing—this is often where the fat and calories accumulate.
3. **Any leftovers from dinner.** See the dinner section below and pick what you would like to eat for lunch.

If you want more guidance on meal planning, I've given you some specific meal plans in Chapter 15 of this book.

Dinner

Dinners can often be the hardest meals to make over. If you have a family, you may feel that your cooking should accommodate their tastes. If you are cooking for one, you often don't want to put in the effort. And furthermore, good food does not have to taste bad. In fact, in Chapter 16 I provide recipes to dispel the myth that mindful eating does not taste delicious. If you are cooking for one, remember that food is an expression of love. Who better to show affection to than yourself? Remember, too, that you're not really cooking just for one since the leftovers will be perfect for breakfast or lunch for the days to come.

The guidelines for healthy dinners are pretty similar to those for healthy lunches. Dinners should include the following components:

- 1 serving of protein (5–6 ounces cooked)
- 1–2 servings of starch
- 2–3 servings of vegetables
- 1 serving of fruit

Here are some dinner ideas that follow these basics:

1. Roasted chicken with a baked sweet potato and salad; fruit salad for dessert
2. Stir-fry with lots of veggies, brown rice, and either chicken, shrimp, or tofu; fruit for dessert
3. Grilled salmon with roasted vegetables and salad; fruit for dessert
4. Grilled pork chop with roasted vegetables and a sweet potato; fruit for dessert
5. Whole-wheat pasta (1 cup at the most) with a homemade pasta sauce with lots of veggies and tomatoes

You'll see from these dinners that the theme is pretty consistent—grilled protein with lots of vegetables. If you want to eat a starch, stick to a fibrous starch such as sweet potatoes, brown rice, or whole-wheat pasta. The point of these makeovers is not to tell you exactly what to eat, but instead to give you a framework with which to make over your own meals. Load up on vegetables—they are high in fibre and nutrients and very low in calories. By far I would argue that vegetables are the healthiest food group around. You would be hard pressed to eat too many. Also, recall from our lunch ideas that your leftovers from dinner can easily serve as lunch (or even breakfast) for the next day. Use these guidelines every day to remodel the meals you eat at home, or follow some specific meal plan ideas in the following chapters.

Eating Out

Eating out is a bit more of a challenge. I am often asked about the best way to eat out healthfully. I am what one would call "a high-maintenance patron"; I always inquire how the food is prepared. I want to know if the fish is grilled or fried. Is there sauce on the vegetables? These details are important when you eat out, and it is perfectly acceptable to ask how the meal is prepared (within reason) and to adjust it to your specifications. Remember, you are paying for this meal, so it should be enjoyable and exactly what you want. Here are some general codes of conduct when eating out:

1. **When it comes to salad, dressing should always be on the side.** Dip your fork in the dressing and then in the salad—you use half the dressing and get all the taste.
2. **If you are having an appetizer, don't have dessert.** If you are having dessert, skip the appetizer. No one needs a three-course meal. Stick with a two-course meal at the most.
3. **Get the bread basket off the table.** You are hungry when you sit down, so it's easy to eat three pieces of bread (that's 300 calories) before your meal arrives.
4. **Only have one unit of alcohol.** A glass of wine or a cocktail, not both. When you are tipsy at dinner you tend to overeat.
5. **If you have a dessert, share it.** Let's be honest, the first bite of something sweet is the best. It's really all downhill after that. There is no need to have an entire dessert all to yourself.
6. **Look up the menu of the restaurant you are going to online.** This allows you to plan your meal choice in

advance and not "impulse purchase" when you get to the restaurant.

7. **Ask for an extra plate to come with your meal.** When the meal arrives, put half of the portion on the extra plate and give it to your server to immediately pack up for you to take home. Most restaurant portions are much bigger than you would ever give yourself, but it's hard to trust yourself to only eat half and take the rest home. Start off the meal by only eating half and you've portion controlled yourself at the beginning of the meal.
8. **Coffee or tea can be as much of a ritual after a meal as dessert can be.** You don't always have to end a meal with a pastry.
9. **A salad makes a perfect appetizer.** Share the main course with your dinner companion and you've economized both your calories and your cash.

Top Tips for Eating Out

Patients often ask me where the best place to eat out is and what are the healthiest choices. Below, I've outlined common types of restaurants and the tips I would recommend when eating at these places.

Steak House

A steak house is probably one of the easiest places to make healthy choices. First of all, all steaks come with measurements—you always know how big your portion is, since you can just ask for the 6-ounce filet. An excellent option at a steak house or at any restaurant is the fish, as long as it is not fried. Ask for the baked potato without anything on it and add your own toppings (just be careful with the amounts). This is a place where you will want to take half your meal home. Steak houses are notorious for offering extra-large portion sizes.

Chinese Food

North American Chinese food restaurants are, in general, not a healthy choice. The meals are often high in added sugars and are usually fried. I tell my patients to both accept their night out at a Chinese food restaurant as a treat for the month and be infrequent with their meals there.

Japanese Restaurants

Stick with sashimi or sushi and watch the portion sizes. A plain green salad is a great starter and a healthy way to fill up. The downfall at Japanese restaurants is, of course, the tempura and deep-fried foods as well as the teriyaki meals, which are full of sugary sauces.

Italian Restaurants

You don't have to shy away from pasta, but a better choice at Italian restaurants would be a meal that involves a grilled protein (fish, chicken, or meat). If you do order the pasta, stick with tomato-based sauces. Cream sauces (such as Alfredo) are high in calories and fat.

American Style

A salad is not always the best choice at an American restaurant. Often they are topped with fried chicken or shrimp. Remember to ask how the meal is prepared before ordering. Stick with the roasted chicken or even a burger with salad instead of fries. You can cut your burger in half and take half home. Now you've still had a burger at a restaurant and it has been a relatively healthy choice.

You can see by this approach that I want you to continue to eat out if it's important to you, but to do so responsibly. Dining out is likely very much a part of your life. Studies show that most North Americans eat out on average three times a week;[76] it would be ideal if you could minimize that to one to two times per week. Regardless, see how you do with a new set of guidelines and tips to work with. Remember, these are meant to be a reference point. Adjust them to your lifestyle and continue to challenge yourself and see how much you can accommodate a healthier approach.

Special Situations

December is an interesting month in my office. In fact, November to January is a time in obesity medicine that brings extra challenges. Patients regularly worry about how they are going to handle the holidays going into December, and by the time January comes around I have a swell of new referrals of people who have made a resolution for the coming year.

This brings me to the concept of special situations; life is full of them. Birthdays, holidays, parties, and weddings are just a few celebrations that deviate from our everyday lives, and they can be hard to navigate in our pursuit of health. There are a variety of events and circumstances that deserve our extra attention when it comes to making a behavioural change, including celebrations, holidays, vacations, and travel. I will discuss each in more detail in the next few sections.

Celebrations

Regardless of the event—a birthday, anniversary, or party—it is crucial that you determine whether the event in question is an extenuating circumstance or an everyday event. Figure out how often parties and birthdays factor into your life. Are you someone who is invited to a kid's birthday party every weekend? Does your job involve a variety of parties and celebrations? Do you have a large extended family such that parties and family dinners are mainstream? You need to determine what your regular life looks like. If parties and birthdays are commonplace, then you need some rules for them. If parties are a rare occurrence and happen less than once a month, I would say enjoy the party (within reason) and view it as an extenuating circumstance and move on.

Scott is forty-three years old and has been seeing me for just over a year. He has lost forty pounds, he exercises every day, and he feels amazing about how far he has come. His life is one big party. Scott has four siblings, and he's married to Lisa, who has three siblings. Together they have five kids of their own. Every weekend there is some sort of family birthday party, wedding, or big dinner. They are a social couple with many reasons to celebrate.

To ask Scott not to engage in these family events is unrealistic and cruel. Celebrations are a part of Scott's life; they are not isolated events that can be completed and contained. Scott easily attends six events per month. His family is big and they like to party, and Scott and Lisa have a big group of friends who also have regular celebrations and events. Scott needs a plan. He has two options: He can minimize the celebrations or he can pick and choose.

Minimize the Celebrations

This idea implies that Scott can "celebrate responsibly." Birthday cakes are commonplace in his life. But does he have to engage in every party to the maximum extent? The goal of this strategy is to ensure that the celebration is treated as an everyday meal with a bit of extra. As such, you will need some rules going into the party to act as a guideline for behaviour:

- Restrict yourself to one alcoholic drink
- No dessert
- Never go back for a second helping
- Try to make healthier choices when possible

Scott tries this strategy for about a month. He makes sure that he goes to the first family party having eaten a nutritious breakfast and lunch. He tells me that he even has a snack sometimes before going to a party and that way if the food is not as nutritious as it could be he eats less and is not as hungry. When cake arrives at his niece's fifth birthday he asks his brother for a piece of fruit. He is really proud of his performance and tries the following week to repeat the behaviour. The event was a cousin's wedding and he tells me that it did not go as well. He had three glasses of wine and found that it impaired his judgment when it came to making healthier choices. Scott brings up a great point: Alcohol, in addition to being empty calories, impairs our ability to "stay on track" when it comes to healthy eating.

Overall Scott found the exercise helpful, but he's looking for other options than just trying to "minimize the damage" at these events. Because there are so many celebrations in his life he would like another set of strategies to use.

Pick and Choose

Is this party *your* birthday, or is it the neighbour's kid's birthday? That is, is it truly a special occasion or one that holds less value? Establish the emotional value for the event and then choose how much you will enjoy it. Furthermore, is this your sister's cooking, which is by far your favourite, or is it dinner at a pizza place where you can easily economize your calories? Not only should you establish what emotional value the event will have, but also establish what kind of enjoyment value the event will have. This is where your sense of food economy will come into play. Is this your mother's Christmas turkey? Or is it your aunt's dried-out meatloaf?

Scott knows all too well which parties in his family have the foods he loves and which ones will be just average from a taste perspective. He also knows which events are coming up a few weeks in advance. I ask him to engage in an exercise where he ranks the events in order of their importance and enjoyment. For example, February looks something like this:

Wife's birthday
Daughter's birthday
Valentine's Day
Two family parties for cousins

Best friend's anniversary party
Three birthdays for kids' friends
Brother's wedding

Scott and I budget that he can pick four events—roughly one per week—that will be special. The rules are that he can't "go crazy" at these events, but that he should enjoy them responsibly. This means he should restrict his alcohol intake to three drinks or less and make sure that the other meals of the day are sound. He should ensure he continues on his regular exercise regimen. Scott picks his four events wisely:

Wife's birthday
Daughter's birthday
Valentine's Day
Brother's wedding

He bases much of his decision on the event's emotional value. For the other six events he is to make sure that he sticks with sound choices and is on extra guard against temptations. What Scott is doing is choosing which events to indulge in and which ones to restrict, so to speak.

The more valuable lesson here is one of practice. As I tell Scott, ironically, the more family events he has, the more practice he will have at managing them. What would once be thought of as a hindrance on his healthy lifestyle should be viewed as an abundance of opportunities to engage his new attitude and to learn where he can make adjustments.

Holidays

Meet Andrea. Andrea has been my patient for about three years, and she has done incredibly well. Her life now looks nothing like it did when she first came to see me. It was a slow process and one that Andrea has worked very hard to achieve and maintain.

Andrea comes to see me in November anxious about the upcoming holidays. She is having twenty-five people to dinner on Christmas and is unsure what to do. She knows that she has to make a feast for her family and needs some guidance. Andrea is not alone. Open a magazine in November and you will undoubtedly see an article about "How to Stay on Your Diet during the Holidays." In addition to having to cook a large meal for her family, Andrea has a variety of work events and social parties to attend. I have several strategies for her.

Regarding her work events and holiday parties, I suggest that Andrea employ one of the two strategies outlined above for celebrations: minimize the celebration or pick and choose. She has six parties in total, but she knows in advance which parties are going to be wonderful culinary experiences. We come up with a plan to have her choose three parties that she will enjoy (responsibly) and three parties that she will go to but be on guard regarding the calories and liquor she consumes.

This brings Andrea to her family dinner. Christmas is the perfect example of the ultimate family dinner. Entertaining in your own home brings with it three typical challenges:

1. The menu
2. Baking
3. Leftovers

The Menu

Because Christmas is at her house this year, I suggest to Andrea that she add a healthy element to her cooking. She has been on this path to health for three years now—what better time to introduce her new way of thinking to her family? I encourage her to look for healthier versions of family favourites. There are a variety of cookbooks available to address healthier holiday options, so I encourage her to have a number of menu items that are "safe" for her.

The key here is to make your menu conform to your new lifestyle. If the dinner is *not* at your house, treat it as you would any celebration: either minimize it or pick and choose. If it is at your house, then make your surroundings conform to suit your new way of life.

Baking

Holiday baking is a big deal for many people. But let's be honest: It's pretty hard to make holiday baking healthier. So don't. The key is to minimize your exposure to it. I hate to be a Grinch, but if you can, don't bake at all.

Sharon is forty-six years old. She normally bakes every Christmas, and her treats are legendary at work. She spends three days baking for Christmas. The problem is that the baking in the house is a temptation for Sharon, and the time she takes to bake is time she is taking away from her family or herself. I highlight for Sharon the cost: the cost of the baking supplies and the cost involved in her time spent baking. We also talk about the cost that the baking will have on her mental well-being, having this kind of temptation in the house. Is all this worth the five minutes of praise she will get from her co-workers for her legendary butter tarts? Perhaps she could take the money she would spend on her baking (a total of $250) and have a day at the spa. She could take one of the extra days she would gain and go skating with her kids and create a new active holiday tradition. What should she bring to her office co-workers instead of baking? I suggest she buy them some pastries from a lovely local bakery. In the end, she'll spend less money *and* have more time.

She is hesitant about making this change, but this year Sharon gives it a try. Turns out she'll never bake again. She has more time for herself and her family, less stress, and less temptation. Her office workers were equally appreciative of the pastries she bought as they were of the ones she baked last year.

If you *must* bake over the holidays, here are some rules to follow:

1. Never keep the baking in the house. Don't freeze the cookies for the kids. They don't need them and you don't want them around.
2. Don't sacrifice your own well-being for baking. Go for a thirty-minute walk before you get into the kitchen. Make sure you have some time for yourself before you become knee deep in ginger snaps.
3. Don't bake while you're hungry.
4. Set yourself a tasting budget. Know before you bake how much you are going to taste and try to stick within it.

Leftovers

People love coming to my house for dinner. Not only do I try to make them feel spoiled beyond belief (if I do say so myself), but they also leave with enough leftovers to last them another meal. It has become a ritual that if you come to my house for dinner, you'll leave with a lunch bag for the next day. I buy those disposable containers at the grocery store and pack them full of a generous serving for as many guests as I can. I leave enough food for my family to last one more meal at the most, and the rest goes out the door. It goes without saying that desserts always leave with a guest.

Leftovers are the perfect parting gift for your dinner guests. It allows them to feel special and you not to feel pressured about having too much food in the house that will tempt your new healthy self.

Back to Andrea. Andrea is going to have twenty-five people at her house for Christmas. She will easily have enough food for thirty-five people. All of the dishes may not be as healthy as she would like, and there will easily be two or three desserts to choose from. Andrea is nervous about having so much food in her house after her guests leave. I suggest that she employ the new leftover rule: Keep enough for one meal for her family and give the rest away.

Andrea gets creative. She buys Chinese takeout boxes in red and green cardboard. She makes the act of giving away leftovers a true event. Three weeks later at her follow-up appointment she is truly gleaming at the success of it all. Her family loved the idea of taking home the extra food and it left her with less stress figuring out what to do with it. The gesture of giving her relatives the leftovers was seen as a gracious and generous act, *and* Andrea respected her new boundaries regarding entertaining and health in her home. As for desserts? Andrea sent the Christmas cake home with her sister and the pumpkin pie home with her in-laws. She glows as she tells me how proud of herself she is.

What strikes me the most about this interaction is how much Andrea has taught herself. This act of trying something new has solidified for her a new strength. No longer does holiday cooking cause her anxiety, because she's been successful in the past with managing things and this has given her the confidence to manage future events.

Here are some of the biggest lessons to learn about holidays:

1. When holiday dinners go terribly wrong, debrief: What would you do next time to make sure that entertaining does not throw off your healthy routine?
2. When holiday dinners go well ask yourself what you have learned and what you are most proud of and continue to repeat that pattern in months to come.

The same principles that apply to Christmas dinner should come into play for other holiday dinners, too. If you are hosting Thanksgiving, take a lesson from Andrea. If you are a guest at someone's house you can celebrate responsibly or take the night off. Thanksgiving comes around one day a year—one day.

Halloween

Halloween is a holiday that deserves individual attention. Halloween was always my favourite holiday as a kid. After all, what kid (chubby or not) does not love getting dressed up and running the streets looking for candy? Back in the 1970s we got apples for Halloween in addition to candy (a shame we can't do that anymore). I remember returning from our trick or treating and my mother having us spill out all the candy on the kitchen table. She let us each pick twenty pieces of candy and the rest went into a big bag that we took to the children's hospital the next day for all the kids who could not go out for Halloween.

It's difficult to be healthy on Halloween. First of all, the Halloween candy inevitably finds its way into the house sometime around the first week in October. I encourage my patients to buy *inedible* Halloween treats. Instead of giving out chocolates or candy (usually your favourite kinds), try giving out Play-Doh or little toys or even toothbrushes. Maybe the kids getting them will hate you, but you will likely hate yourself more for eating an entire bag of leftover candy.

If you must buy candy for Halloween, buy it on October 31. Make sure you empty the candy bowl by the time the evening is done. If it's lights out by 10 P.M., the kid who comes to your house at 9:45 is the luckiest child alive, because he or she will get whatever candy is left in the bowl.

Finally, if you have kids that are bringing their own loot into the house, take a lesson from what my mother did with us. Have the kids count out ten to twenty candies and send the rest to the food bank, or take it into work for your co-workers, or yes, even put it in the garbage. An even better thought? Have your kids call on twenty houses then take them for a really long walk after. Just a thought.

Vacations

Our lives should have moments of escape. I want you to enjoy your holidays and get away from your everyday life. That being said, there is no reason why your holidays need to be an escape from your healthy lifestyle. Your vacations should be part of your healthy lifestyle, not a return to the unhealthy way things used to be.

Here are some strategies for how to stay on track during times of travel and vacations. Many of these scenarios can be applied to the business traveller as well.

The Plane

My friends laugh at me on a plane. I do travel a lot for work, and like a Boy Scout, I always come prepared. First, I pack a meal for the plane. This prevents me from being hungry mid-flight and having to buy the less healthy snacks available for purchase on most airlines. My plane meals look pretty much like my usual lunches. If you forget to pack a meal for the plane, most airports sell healthy options such as a salad to go or fruit and yogurt. Make healthier choices and start your travel off on the right note.

The Hotel

Almost every hotel will allow you to rent a bar fridge for your room. The cost is usually an extra $5 per day and well worth the expense. When you arrive at your hotel, ask the front desk staff where the nearest grocery store is and make a trip to stock up on some "healthy essentials," such as fresh fruit, cut vegetables, and low-fat yogurt. You can even buy some items to make a healthy breakfast or lunch. One of the best ideas on holiday is to ensure that at least one of your daily meals is not eaten in a restaurant but prepared by you in the hotel. The easiest meal for this is often breakfast, and you can use the techniques we've already talked about—instant oatmeal or a protein bar is a perfect and fast breakfast. Let's be frank: You don't eat three meals a day in a restaurant at home, so don't do it on your vacation. You will save calories just by making one meal a day in your hotel room.

Exercise

Being on holiday does not mean being sedentary. In fact, vacations are the perfect time to be more active. Every hotel has a gym—use it. Set a time of day and make sure you get in a certain amount of exercise. Furthermore, you can find other opportunities to be active on vacation. Get to the airport thirty minutes early, check in, then walk around the airport before getting on the plane. Once you've arrived in your vacation destination go for a walk. You will be surprised at how much more you will love the city you are visiting just by walking in it.

Deviating from the everyday does not have to push you off track. For most of us travelling for work is the norm and having family over for dinner and celebrations is a common occurrence. If these "special situations" are in fact a part of your everyday life find a way to make your healthy habits translate to these situations. If you travel for work, bring your healthy habits with you on the road. Pack a lunch for the plane, walk the airport before you take off and when you land, and have a bar fridge in your hotel room.

The key message here is to use your life as your classroom and learn how to make it healthier. Decide from the outset if your "special situations" are really unique, or if they are, in fact, regular occurrences. If the latter is true, you need to treat them as everyday opportunities to learn how to be healthier.

12

Embrace the Suck: How to Be Good at Being Bad

As human beings we learn by making mistakes. When we make changes in our lives, mistakes will inevitably happen. How do we turn those mistakes into learning opportunities? How do we get comfortable with the mistake itself and see the lesson behind it?

Weight loss and lifestyle change is no different. How do we learn from past diets to shape our dieting future? It's quite simple: We embrace the suck. What I mean is that we embrace that which we are bad at in order to get better. By doing so, we turn our greatest weakness into our greatest strength. I've met thousands of people who lost weight successfully and then gained it back—it really is a devastating process. There is the saying "it is better to have loved and lost than never to have loved at all," but that simply isn't true for weight loss. In fact, both physically and mentally, it is *not* better to have lost and then gained than never to have lost at all.

When I met Natalie she was, in her words, at her "lowest point." She was twenty-eight years old and had been on every diet available. She had spent more days than not on any given diet. She had tried both conventional and online programs; she had bought prepackaged foods and meal delivery programs; she had a personal nutritionist and a personal trainer.

Each time, Natalie would lose weight. She would spend months on a program and then fall off track. Sometimes the slip was gradual—she would slowly start to "cheat" (her words, not mine) and indulge in foods that were not on her given program. One indulgence would lead to several and before long she was off her program. Sometimes Natalie's slip was sudden. When she was twenty-six her sister got engaged. It was a destination wedding and Natalie was determined to lose weight for the wedding. She tried a starvation program where she ate 800 calories per day and got special "vitamin shots." Natalie lost sixty pounds in six months. She went to the wedding in Mexico, and it was fabulous; she looked and felt amazing. While there she gained five pounds in a week. Six months after the wedding, Natalie had gained all of her weight back.

She begins to cry as she tells me of her struggle from one cycle of weight loss and gain to another. I spend time talking with Natalie about what she learned from the programs that did *not* work for her. What did she take away about her patterns of behaviour? What insights does she have into her behaviour? Why didn't the programs work? Natalie makes a list of the five things that she has learned from her dieting disasters:

1. I can't do extreme diets. I hate programs that force me to give up everything.
2. I need something that still lets me have a life while I'm watching what I'm eating.
3. I like to exercise. I like how strong I feel when I am active. It's not a problem for me to do some sort of activity every day.
4. I'm not very good at keeping track of what I eat. I do okay keeping a food diary for a while, and then I fall off track and spiral out of control. Then I feel guilty about not having kept a food diary and so I let things slide even further.

5. I tend to beat myself up when I fall off track on a program. I get really mad at myself and really angry but I seem powerless to do something about it. Nothing anyone says is worse than the voice in my head.

Natalie is stuck in a pattern where her mistakes drive her away from a learning opportunity because she is afraid to fail. Enter the concept I call "embrace the suck." This is where you accept your misgivings in order to learn and move forward. Natalie needs to embrace the suck: She must accept that she has to be bad at something before she can get good at it.

Human beings often react to their misgivings in one of two ways: We either shy away from the things we aren't good at, or we repeatedly make the same mistakes over and over again and therefore continue to fall short in those areas. But what if instead of avoiding the mistakes or repeating them we just accepted our misgivings and moved on?

For instance, I can't play an instrument. Sure, I had the requisite piano lessons that many children have, but I never really stuck with it. I lack the patience and the focus necessary to sit and practise regularly to become a master at an instrument. Don't get me wrong, I am very patient and focused in other areas of my life, but when it comes to learning piano or guitar, I just don't have it. So I stand back and accept that the piano is just not for me, and I have learned not to think too much of it. It's not personal—it does not say anything about my character. When I admit that I don't have what it takes to be a concert pianist it does not make me sad or disenchanted with my life. "I'm good at other things," I think, and move on.

When it comes to weight loss many of us have tried and fallen off track. Maybe we lack the patience in that moment or the focus in another. It's not personal—this is not a flaw in our character, but rather who we are. Instead of chastising ourselves, why not change our perspective and learn from our limitations?

Natalie admits that her decade of dieting has taught her that severely restrictive programs prohibit her from having a normal life. And because she wants a normal life she can't follow these programs for long. Instead of making the change to find a program that meets her life's demands she chastises herself over and over again for not being able to conform to that which she already admits is impossible for her. The solution is right in front of her eyes: She needs to acknowledge her own limitations and instead of being ashamed of them, adjust her next healthy change to meet those demands.

Natalie's next program should *not* be severe. It should be one that allows her to have celebrations with friends and family (within reason), but affirms for her that this is who she is. She has to let go of the idea that she must be denied to lose weight. Severe dieting may work for some (I'd love to meet those people), but it certainly does not work for Natalie. If she keeps attempting the same pattern over and over again all she can look forward to is disappointment and self-blame.

Natalie thinks she needs to learn discipline to succeed. She thinks she needs to learn how to just "suck it up" and stick to a diet—she could not be more wrong. I know that Natalie needs to learn patience and forgiveness; she needs to forgive herself for her own limitations. So she can't stick to a program that only allows her to eat 800 calories a day—who can? It's a challenge at best and I would argue an unhealthy one. She needs to see this inability to starve herself as a blessing, not a curse.

Instead, Natalie should focus on the positive things she has learned thus far. She needs to focus on the things that she is good at. For example, she has learned that she likes to exercise. She can use that information to plot out an exercise plan that will play to her strengths and give her something positive, both physically and mentally, to feel good about.

Finally, Natalie needs to be patient. Weight loss and healthy living are an everyday process without an end. She needs to abandon the idea of "destination dieting." I explain to her that it is no wonder that she fell off track every time she went on a program. She always dieted with a specific "destination" in mind. Whether it was a family wedding, a holiday, or some other event, she always went on a program with her eye on a specific "due date." Once the event took place it was as though there was an alarm that went off in her brain saying, "Yup, we're done." She needs to move beyond this idea that there are markers of success and see that getting healthier is a fluctuating and never-ending process.

"So how will I know when I am there? When I've reached my goal?" she asks.

"You'll evaluate it on a daily basis, just like you do everything else in your life. Some days are good, others not so much. You go to bed and wake up the next morning and pledge to be better," I respond.

"When did you realize that you had reached your goal?" she asks.

I respond with my usual answer to this question: "Any day now."

In 2009 I decided that I was going to learn how to "clip in" on my bicycle. I wanted to get those special pedals and special shoes for my bicycle that allow you to literally clip into the pedal and be attached to the bike. The advantage of this is that you pedal more effectively; the disadvantage is that you can forget to clip out of the pedal and fall off your bike.

I was determined. I had owned my bike for six months and had ridden it every day. I was ready to take it to the next level and learn to clip in. I had the special pedals placed on my bike and bought the special shoes. I took my bike to a grassy park area and began learning how to clip in and out of the pedals. I fell eighteen times. I took my bike home and put it on one of those bike trainers and I practised clipping in and out. I even had the pedals changed to a different pedal that would be easier to clip in and out of. I was terrible at it—I just plain sucked at slipping in and out of my bike pedals, regardless of what I did. But I persevered.

I remember people telling me at the time that I was crazy. I was crazy for continuing to try to learn to do something that I was failing at. I had fallen off my bike a total of eighteen times, and yet I was still ready for the nineteenth fall. My tenacity, my dog-with-a-bone attitude, may have been my greatest weakness or it may have been my greatest strength. I was stubborn beyond reproach and I would not give up—I would master this skill.

Sure I almost killed myself a few times, but I learned. I could easily have switched the pedals back to the usual ones and abandoned the process entirely. Instead I remembered that I had to be bad at something before I could get good at it. I sucked at clipping in and out of the bike pedals, but I had to embrace the fact that I sucked to move forward and get better. Now some years later, clipping in and out of my bike is second nature for me. The lesson here is more than just one about a bad cyclist trying to be a better one; it is a lesson in the value of humility: You have to be bad before you can get better. You have to embrace the suck. When you see the value in the fall, only then are you ready for the climb.

I tell this to my patients each time they try to embark on a new lifestyle change. They are scared because they have been so terrible at it in the past. And yet they persevere. Their tenacity becomes both what they see as their greatest weakness and what I see as their greatest strength. They have tried so many programs in the past and feel like a failure. I, on the other hand, see their perseverance and continued commitment to change as their greatest accomplishment. They are still in the game, and that is something indeed.

How do you continue in this way? How do you persevere despite unknown odds and unknown values? You embrace the things you feel you lack the skills to do well and learn to get better at them. You reflect upon what your weaknesses are and see them for the hidden strengths they might be.

Stop Asking Why

We are creatures of habit. We really do engage in routine, whether it is healthy or not. For some reason it works for us; regardless of the motivator, we just do it ... over and over and over again. It does not matter if the pattern is a healthy one or an unhealthy one; it does not matter if the pattern is convenient or inconvenient, easy or challenging. The key is the pattern itself more than its descriptors. Ask most people why they do certain things and they will often give you the answer "Because I do."

Sure, we'd love to know why things happen. I see it all the time: "Doctor, *why* did this happen? Why can't I lose weight? Why do I keep making the same mistakes over and over again?" Here's the thing: "Why" questions don't have answers. Questions that begin with "why" are often the ones we say looking up at the heavens in complete disbelief. The most common misconception of any weight-loss program is that you must figure out *why* you do the things you do in order to fix them. And that works for some people. Some of us are able to determine the exact root of the problem, but I would argue that we often discover the cause by finding the cure.

Let me introduce you to Lea. Lea is one great lady. I know I should not have favourites, but at least I am honest. Lea is forty-six years old and had been overweight since her early twenties. She has been my patient for almost three years. To date, Lea has lost over a hundred pounds. It has been a long process, and in fact, Lea will tell you that her dieting history dates back over twenty years. My admiration for Lea goes well beyond her hundred-pound weight loss, though. No doubt she is an inspiration to anyone who meets her: She has faced her disease head-on and has successfully challenged the status quo. But beyond that, Lea is a perfect example of what happens when you stop asking *why* and start asking *what*.

Lea had been on every program imaginable. Each program began the same way: She started with fervour. But like many all-or-nothing dieters something would happen and Lea would fall off track. She would be challenged to resume her healthy habits at the same intensity, and she would mentally beat herself up for her inability to get back on track.

Lea is a psychologist by trade. Every day she helps others come to terms with the "why" of their own lives. So she sought counselling for her own pattern of dieting. She tells me that she spent years in therapy trying to get to the root of why she wavered on a variety of programs. Sure, she found some answers, but she tells me quite pragmatically that those answers did not necessarily change her behaviour. "You don't figure out why you are heavy and then a light bulb goes on and it's all better," she says matter-of-factly. "I'm not sure when it happened, but I just decided that I'd done all the therapy that was helpful. But now I had to *do* something to change what I had learned about myself. I could either accept that this was who I was and this was the way it was going to be, or I could make a change in my everyday life and see what happened." See what I mean? Go Lea.

Just because you know why you behave the way you do with food and exercise does not necessarily mean your problem will be fixed instantly. I think people are conditioned to think that because we know "why" something occurs, we can fix it. That is not the case. Figure out the "why" or don't. But once you do, find something to do differently. *Do not dwell on the why.*

By no means do I intend to discourage you from seeking counselling to better understand your current patterns of behaviour. I am not saying that the "why" is unimportant; what I am saying is that understanding why you do certain things is *not* a prompt for change, and it is also *not* necessary. Feel free to figure out why you behave a certain way toward food and exercise, but don't think of it as a mandatory step to change. Maybe you will discover that there is a deep-seated issue, or maybe you will find out that it is just habit. Either way, whatever you find searching for the "why," you will need to establish a plan of action. In other words, once you figure out the "why" (if indeed you do), get yourself a "what," meaning figure out what to do.

Here's an interesting exercise. Ask yourself the following questions:

Why	What
Why do I have no control over certain foods?	What can I do with foods that have "power" over me?
Why do I eat beyond fullness?	What will I do when I am full?
Why don't I eat better?	What can I do to eat better?
Why don't I exercise more?	What can I do to exercise more?
Why can't I be healthier?	What is preventing me from being healthier?

You can see that the "why" column allows for in-depth questions that may or may not have answers. The "what" column, on the other hand, leaves you with a plan of attack—"what" questions give you a place to start. I tell my patients all the time to stick with questions that begin with "what" and you will have a place to start. Interestingly, I suspect that the more you progress through this healthy process, the further along you will be to gaining a key as to *why* certain things are the way that they are.

Lea spent years in therapy, and perhaps she gained some greater insight into herself, her eating, and her obesity. But it was not until she began changing her patterns of behaviour toward food and exercise that she began to do something about those insights. Lea will be the first to tell you that she learned more about why she was obese by losing weight than she did in her counsellor's office. Isn't that always the case? When we find our way home, don't we learn more about how we got lost in the first place?

Our behaviours are a reflection of who we are and what we think. Your thoughts become your language, your language becomes part of your actions, and your actions become a part of who you are. So why can't our actions shape what we think and reflect who we are and how we communicate? I absolutely think they can.

There are two schools of thought in psychology in this regard. The first school of thought suggests that we have an inspiration or a prompt that in turn moves us toward a certain action.[77] The other school of thought maintains that actions prompt our inspiration and our thoughts, which in turn continue to promote our actions. In effect, you do something and it motivates you to continue doing it or to do something else. In case you have not guessed, I'm a fan of the second school of thought. When it comes to weight loss, I'm not sure what the inspiration was that woke me up and prompted me to lose more than half my body weight, but I do know what actions were involved. I also know that these very actions have become a part of who I am and, as such, continue to motivate me to keep on the path.

Lea had learned the language in her therapy sessions; she'd figured out the key to who she was. But it was not until she changed her actions to reflect that knowledge that she truly healed and became the person she was meant to be. This is the key message: Lea's actions did more to establish her sense of who she was than the years of trying to figure out her motivation.

If we return to the concept of "why" and "what" we can see how actions can be a powerful tool to reshaping how we think. To this day I'm really not sure *why* I weighed 320 pounds. Sure, I was always predisposed genetically and physiologically to being overweight and obese, but to stop there means that I am powerless to change my habits; to stop there means I am just a kid with a birthday cake wishing my weight away. But it was when I blew out the candles and starting doing something about it that I really made my wish come true. When I started asking myself "what" I could do to be healthier was when the actions came pouring in.

So from this day forward, change the question from "Why am I unhealthy today?" to "What can I do today to be healthier tomorrow?" Simply asking the right question will give you a list of things to do, a place to start—in short, a blueprint for change.

13

What to Do When You Get Derailed

We all have bad days, and even bad weeks. What we do in those moments often defines who we are, but it does not have to. What if we used those times of derailment to learn something empowering? What if those moments became ones that did not weaken our resolve, but ones that strengthened our knowledge base?

I've mentioned before that as we move through this process we need to shift the normal. We need to establish certain patterns of behaviour that are the "new normal." The problem is that when we have a setback, we often don't have a new behaviour that reflects the new normal. We turn to our old patterns during these times, perhaps out of desperation, to re-establish the normal once again.

Sandy comes to see me. She was, in her words, "doing so well and then it all fell apart." Sandy has been my patient for almost six months. She definitely has a component of emotional eating and was inactive when we first met. Sandy also used to drink a significant amount of her calories—she loved juice and ginger ale and had them both daily. We spent her first month with me getting her off the liquid sugar and onto an exercise plan. She has spent the last few months identifying her emotional triggers and her food cues and working to adjust her relationship with food in these circumstances. Sandy had a strategy going into Christmas and was able to manage the holiday season with success. She is very proud of the way she navigated a variety of holiday parties. Sandy has a treadmill at home that she now uses for forty-five minutes every day, which is her bare minimum. When she is not able to do forty-five minutes at a time she goes on the treadmill for twenty minutes at least, and she usually finds that twenty minutes into her walk she feels great and wants to continue.

All was going so well in "Sandyland," and then she got the flu. It began with her kids and spread like wildfire through the house. Everyone was sick—it was nasty. She could not exercise (bare minimum or not) for more than three weeks. For the first week all she wanted to do was stay in bed and drink juice and ginger ale, finding comfort in her old habits. Then came the emotional downfall. She felt bad about drinking her calories and felt that all her hard work was being flushed down the toilet. She was sick and she felt horrible, both physically and mentally. Physically, Sandy had the flu and she wanted comfort foods. She began healthfully with soups, but quickly moved on to pastas with cream sauce and cream soups. Emotional triggers pushed her toward the pantry and Sandy indulged. After all, Sandy was sick and Sandy "deserved it."

It only took ten days for Sandy to return to her old habits. She tells me that one of her biggest triggers was not being able to exercise. Feeling unwell and not being able to get out of bed put her in the wrong frame of mind, so she brought her old "comfort foods" into the house and went through them with abandon. Sandy sits in my office and talks about the experience, almost disconnected.

"I almost did not recognize myself," she says in a bit of disbelief. "I was on a pity party and I could not make it end. For almost a month I ate whatever I wanted and drank all the juice and sugar I could. It began slowly and then snowballed. I feel like I'm back where I started from."

"How are you right now?" I ask, trying to get a sense of where we are in the process.

"Well, I've started back on the treadmill, but I've easily gained five pounds."

Sandy and I discuss how she is by no means back at the beginning. For one thing, she has already tried to get herself back on track before coming in to see me. For another thing, she has acknowledged where she has gone wrong and has started to break down the details of where the wheels fell off the car, so to speak. This event is *not* a failure but a learning opportunity, so Sandy and I talk about how she can get back on track.

To learn from it, we need to examine what Sandy did this past month. Quite simply, what she did was turn to her old habits because that was the default pattern of behaviour that she had used so often in the past. Sandy knows what to do when she is well; she's spent months establishing the normal for that. When she got sick, though, it was her very own special situation, one that she had not planned for. As such she turned to her old patterns of behaviour because that is all the experience she had to draw upon. When that behaviour did not make her feel better, Sandy got desperate. She was terrified that she was now fully back to the old ways, so she reached out for a maladaptive method to re-establish the new normal.

What Sandy does not realize, sitting in my office, is that she does not have to scramble to get back on track. She just needs to establish a behaviour plan for instances like this. I ask Sandy what she learned from this setback: "I learned that even though I thought I was fixed in the juice department, I'm not. I used my illness as an excuse to drink my juice and ginger ale. When it comes to the sugar drinks, I'm still really vulnerable."

"What would you do differently next time?" I ask.

"I would not even have them in the house. In a way it was good to see how susceptible I am to sugar drinks. I know better for next time."

"What's the plan for the next time you get the flu?"

"Vitamin C tablets and diet ginger ale. Lots of sugar-free fluids or just water."

Sandy's lessons are universal. Our new habits and new lifestyle have become the "new normal." The issue with this new normal is that it lacks the wealth of experience that our "old normal" had. As such, we need to have these unforeseen circumstances—these so-called falls from grace—so that we can stock our armory with lessons and experiences upon which to draw in future times.

Research has shown that longevity is one of the key predictors of weight-loss success.[78] People who have lost a significant amount of weight over long periods of time and have kept the weight off for long periods are more likely to achieve long-term weight-loss success. The longer you keep the weight off, the longer you will keep it off. This, of course, seems pretty logical, but there is also a lesson here. From a physiological perspective, losing weight slowly and keeping it off gives your brain and body chemistry sufficient time to adjust to the new biochemical lay of the land. From a behavioural perspective, you have allowed for a sufficient amount of life's events, both joyous and otherwise, to occur and teach you lessons that you need to learn to keep your new habits. You have had opportunities for derailment and may even have fallen off track a few times. You have had the opportunity to learn how to adjust your new way of life to meet the usual demands of others around you. The key to remember is that your old patterns of behaviour may have not changed along with you. Sandy has given up sugar drinks, eats properly, and exercises regularly. But Sandy still lives in the same world where less than a year ago her behaviours were much different than they are today. Furthermore, Sandy still lives in a world where she gets the flu every now and then.

The Derailers

In my experience a variety of events, both positive and negative, can cause a setback. The three most common derailers are as follows:

1. Sickness, flu, or other short-term illness
2. Injury
3. Feeling great

Sickness and Flu

The average North American gets two colds per year, and the average cold lasts one to two weeks.[79] Let's put this in perspective: If you can't exercise for four weeks out of the year, settle down. Remember that when you are feeling better you may not be able to get back to the previous intensity you were at right away. No worries—start again with the twenty to thirty minutes you began with and work your way up to where you were.

Injuries

It's key that we talk for a moment about injuries. We all get injured, and now I am asking you to get more active, so you are bound to hurt something. Furthermore, some of you already have arthritis in one joint or another.

Injuries can derail even the most focused among us. The key here is to have a back-up plan. If you can't walk on a treadmill, go to water aerobics. The pool is closed for cleaning for a month? Try a home exercise video that is low impact. How about a stationary bike? When you choose an exercise make sure you always have a Plan B. This also allows for times when the weather is not cooperating.

Last year I tore my hamstring, so running was out of the question. I was training for a triathlon and I was devastated. It was in those moments, going through physiotherapy and rehab, that I realized I had to take a lesson from myself. What would I say to a patient in the same situation? Simple: I would tell her to focus on swimming and cycling and the exercising she *could* do without pain while her hamstring was healing. I would tell her to remember that this happens and having an alternative form of exercise is mandatory. I needed to focus on what I *could* do and not dwell on what I could *not* do.

A back-up plan to both nutritional choices and exercise is key in this process. It gives us an alternative that often may be more effective and enjoyable than the initial plan. As for me? It turns out I like cycling and swimming even more than I like running. I am slowly back at running nonetheless, but having other activities to choose from and rotate into my training schedule has allowed me to minimize further risk of injury and to experiment with other forms of exercise. My torn hamstring forced me to think outside the current possibilities, and I found that there was a whole other world of exercise waiting for me to enjoy.

Feeling Great

Sometimes we get "cocky." A little success can derail us as much as it can motivate us further. We make some changes, the scale responds, and we figure "I got this." A celebration or a vacation comes around and suddenly there is no need to adhere to our new healthy patterns of behaviour.

We feel great and that will be enough to ward off the old habaits. And suddenly almost seamlessly we're back into our previous patterns of behaviour and we almost don't know how it happened.

Getting Back on Track

When we do fall off track in the new normal, we strive to return to that new normal but our skills and our response, emotional and otherwise, reflect some of our old patterns of behaviour. There are a variety of reactions that occur in this instance:

1. We get desperate.
2. We come from a negative place.
3. We doubt our abilities to get back on track.
4. We give up.

Reaction #1: We Get Desperate

The solution here is to resist the quick fix. When people fall off track, they often get desperate and look for a "quick fix" to "shock" the system back into place. I have seen this all too many times. People turn to starvation programs or grapefruit diets—quick fixes that they feel are needed as a means to get them back into their previous program.

Often, people's reaction to desperation is to make terrible decisions. We see this in life, in business, and in lifestyle management. When you make decisions rooted in anxiety, fear, or distraction you don't make good decisions. For one thing, you can't see the long-term repercussions of your decisions because they are clouded in the desperation. The biggest issue with these decisions is that your new healthy path is a slow one. It was derived from a place of forgiveness and positivity; it was optimistic and it allowed for slow, methodical changes. Turning to an opposite "quick fix" as a means of helping you get back to that positive place is ludicrous.

Some years ago I sat on the admissions committee to my alma mater, McMaster School of Medicine. An applicant once asked me about the process of admissions. She was a vibrant, twenty-one-year-old woman who was applying to nursing as a "stepping stone" to medicine. I asked her outright, "Do you want to be a nurse?"

"No, of course not. I want to be a doctor. But I figure this will get me in the door, right?"

"Wrong. If you want to be a doctor, apply to medical school. If you want to be a nurse, apply to nursing. Don't potentially take a spot away from a future nurse and don't waste four years of your life in a school you don't want to be in." Yeah, I was blunt, but it is one of my terrible habits in life.

The point of this comparison is that if you want a healthy approach to food and exercise, don't start from an unhealthy place. If you want to achieve true health and positivity regarding your relationship with food and exercise, start on a process that will allow for this. Sandy had been in a place that she wanted to get back to. How she does that is to engage in the steps that got her there in the first place.

Resist the quick fix and the desperation. It likely has not worked for you many times in the past, so don't repeat your same mistakes in the hopes that somehow, magically, this time they will be made right.

Reaction #2: We Come from a Negative Place

The solution here is to be kind, because people respond well to kindness. Sandy's initial instinct was to beat herself up emotionally because she was mad at herself for her downfall. She was harsh in her self-talk. This is a natural response to what we perceive as failure. The problem with this response is that it is not very effective in getting people what they want. Overwhelmingly, studies show that students learn better in an encouraging environment. Biochemically the studies show that the brain is more effective in its performance when it does *not* feel threatened.[80]

When I was about eight years old my parents decided to give me piano lessons. My teacher's name was Mrs. Katchinsky. She has likely long since passed away, and I know we should not speak ill of the dead, and further, I am sure Mrs. Katchinsky meant well. However, she single-handedly made me hate piano lessons. She would give me sheets of music to practise and play, which I would take home and practise. When I returned to her home the following Thursday night, I would sit in her dimly lit living room in front of her Steinway grand piano (it was a glorious piece of art that I loved to play), but every time I made a mistake on the homework sheets she would hit my knuckles with her hand. No, there were no bruises, don't get excited; even though today children's services would no doubt be involved, it was the 1970s and this was viewed as "normal." Rest assured I turned out okay—I just hated Mrs. Katchinsky and I hated piano lessons.

The point is, I did not learn well when I felt threatened—all I learned was to hate piano lessons. I put up with Mrs. Katchinsky for a while and was a pretty decent piano player, but I hated every minute of it. About three years later I switched teachers and met Mrs. Spencer, the piano teacher's equivalent of Julie Andrews. She was elegant and fabulous. She loved music and *loved* teaching music. Mrs. Spencer let me play whatever I wanted; she let me improvise and pick the music. She even encouraged her students to sing along if we wanted. Most importantly, when I made a mistake on the keys, I would stop to apologize and she would pretend that it was just a part of the piece.

"Why'd you stop?" she would ask.

"I screwed up,"

"Who doesn't?" she laughed. "Keep playing."

Mrs. Spencer may not have made me a better pianist, but she made me love the piano again. For an eight-year-old who was never going to be a concert pianist she gave me the best gift ever: She taught me that we learn from a place of ease and kindness far better than from a place of shame and regret.

Forgiveness is key in this process. You fell off track—welcome to the human race. Stop hitting yourself on the knuckles and move on. Instead of beating yourself up, make a list of the things you learned along the way and try to find ways to problem solve through them for the next time.

Reaction #3: We Doubt Our Abilities to Get Back on Track

The solution here is to practise, practise, practise. Studies in positive psychology and learning show that we can change how our brain functions just by repeatedly engaging in a new task. Functional MRI studies on people who have lost their sight at birth show that after learning to read Braille, the visual word form area (VWFA) expands over time. What is even more amazing is that we use this VWFA in sighted reading as well.[81] Furthermore, people who have been blind from birth and those who have normal sight both use the VWFA to read Braille. Braille has only been around for about 200 years, whereas visual reading has been around for about

5500 years. Could it be that because our brains did not have time to adapt to Braille and blindness it just used its regular reading centres for a different purpose? This study and others like it show that we can change how our brains perceive certain situations, but still use what we have to make it work. Furthermore, the evidence suggests that we do so in a much more effective way if we approach this process from a positive place.

It's natural to doubt your abilities. This is likely not the first time you have started a program and fallen off track—your dieting history has come back to haunt you. How will this time be different? Through attitude and actions, that's how. You can't just will this to be a positive experience, but you can engage in the actions outlined in the previous chapters and highlighted below to get back on track.

Reaction #4: We Give Up

This one is simple: don't. It sounds pretty easy and perhaps a bit pedestrian, but if you never give up there will always be a possibility. I tell my patients all the time, "I can't treat an empty chair." What you see as a failure is purely a learning opportunity. If you walk away, you lose out on both the learning opportunity and the possibility of turning the whole situation around. Just don't give up. Even if this book does not work for you, try something else. This is your health we're talking about, and everyone deserves to be healthy. Whatever you do, don't give up.

The message here is clear: Resist the temptation for a quick fix to get you back on track. Instead, reflect upon the situation and the triggers that allowed you to fall off track in the first place. Retrace your steps. Approach this setback from a place of positivity and allow yourself forgiveness for the fall so that you can move forward. Never doubt your abilities to move forward and regardless of what happens, NEVER GIVE UP.

So here we are, ready to move past your setback. As I see it, you have one of three options:

1. **Start back at the beginning.** Everyone deserves a "do over" once in a while, so simply start over. Interestingly, Sandy thought she was back at the beginning until she realized how much different she was even six months into the process. You are likely not back where you started emotionally or even behaviourally, and two weeks of Sandy's indulgence was not going to undo six months of daily commitment. That being said, she began back at the beginning by keeping a food diary and exercising twenty minutes every day. In short, she went back to her basic rules and began again.
2. **Pick up where you left off.** What were you doing, exercise- and food-wise, when the meteor struck? Were you exercising forty-five minutes every day? Were you off sugar drinks entirely? Well, there's no reason why you can't just pick up where you left off. This is definitely a harder option to entertain, and many people prefer to start back again slowly. That being said you may want to see if you can realistically pick up where you left off.
3. **Retrace your steps and use the tools that work for you.** This is key. Sandy found that her rules and her food diary were hard-wired tools that helped her stay on track in the past. So return to what works for you. Yes, it will be challenging, but you already know that it is effective in the long term.

After you've gotten yourself back on track (because you will), you need to plan for future setbacks. The key here is to remember that you *learned* something and you know what you can do differently next time. Setbacks can be very powerful in a positive way if we learn to use their teachings.

Jenny is a mother to a four-year-old little girl and an elementary school teacher. She has been my patient for about three years and has lost fifty pounds and kept it off. Two summers ago, Jenny had a huge setback. She is someone who does very well with structure, and the school year is the perfect time for her to be organized. She loves schedules and has incorporated exercise into her schedule. As you can also imagine, Jenny *loves* keeping a food diary (no, really, she does!). It speaks to her strength of being organized. But two summers ago she was without a schedule and everything fell apart. She lost track of her exercise schedule and her food diary. Ironically, too much free time did not allow for the structure that she needed in her daily life.

Jenny gained eight pounds that summer. She came back to see me in September in tears. I let her have a good cry and then we got to work. What I highlighted for Jenny was how the summer had effectively shown her what she was made of. "You know what you need to stay on track," I said. "Most people search their whole lives for the key to the kingdom and you've got it figured out."

Jenny needed to see that what she perceived as a failure was really her key to the kingdom: Jenny realized how important structure and planning are to her success and well-being. Now, two years later, Jenny goes into every summer with a summer schedule. She plans daily leisure activities for her holidays, which allows her to schedule in her exercise and plays to her strength. Jenny has spent two summers since then on track with the full knowledge that although it might seem unconventional for others, she needs to plan her holidays for them to be truly relaxing for her.

Setbacks are going to happen. The key is to use them to your advantage and not allow them to be permanently detrimental. The most successful among us in any endeavour will often tell you that they learned more from their failures than from their successes. If this is truly the case, open your eyes and look forward to the educational experiences ahead.

14

Staying the Course

There is a great deal of science behind dieting, but the psychology of this process is a different story entirely. We start program after program expecting that this time will be different—this time we will lose that elusive amount of weight. Daniel Gilbert is a world-renowned psychologist and an expert on happiness.[82] A few years ago I watched a TED talk given by Dr. Gilbert, which I have watched many times since to keep the message fresh in my memory. In it, Gilbert talks about the Dutch philosopher Bernoulli and his famous equation for happiness and success from 1738:

$$\text{Expected Value} = \text{Odds of Gain} \times \text{Value of Gain}$$

Basically, Bernoulli's equation states that the expected value of an experience is the product of the odds of gaining a given item multiplied by the value of the item itself. For example, we assign a value to any experience that we have based on the value of the experience itself and also based on the chance of gaining that experience.

Let's take medical school as an example. For anyone, getting into medical school does have a certain value to it. For me it was definitely a product of the chance of me getting in and the value of being a doctor someday. As someone applying to medicine in 1993, I, like my fellow students, had calculated the odds. I knew, for example, that the McMaster School of Medicine had approximately 4000 applicants each year for about a hundred spots. I knew the odds of the gain, and I assumed the value of someday being a doctor would be worth it. As an obesity physician many years later I calculate odds regularly. I assess patients at regular visits and wonder if the breakthrough they need with their health will come this time. Will this interaction be the one that makes the impact?

How do you calculate the odds when it comes to weight-loss success? Can you calculate odds when it comes to human behaviour? More importantly, *should* we calculate odds of success when it comes to something as individual and personal as the pursuit of health? In pondering this, I could not help but wonder if Bernoulli's equation could be applied to people trying to lose weight.

First, what is the value of losing weight? The value we assign to this endeavour is unique for every individual. People's motivations for weight loss are so numerous and so diverse. I surveyed my patients over a one-week period with one question: Why do you want to lose weight? Here were some of the answers:

- To be happier
- To be less alone
- To be healthier
- To get off medications
- To live longer
- To wear nicer clothes
- To be included
- To belong
- To feel better
- To not be in pain

As you can appreciate, these are some pretty high values assigned to the concept of weight loss—there is much to be gained by this process.

Bernoulli's equation states that we have to calculate the odds of achieving a specific item. We can assign value to an experience by calculating our odds of attaining that experience and the value of that experience itself. But if we break it down even further, one of the greatest problems with weight loss and our expectations of weight loss is that we have an unrealistic value of what weight loss will bring to our lives, and furthermore it is next to impossible to calculate the odds of attaining it. Most people who have tried to lose weight in the past have been unsuccessful; they have a negative association with weight loss because they feel they have failed in the past. Therefore, they can't calculate its possibility because it is already unattainable.

We've all heard a variation of the story about a kid who, at the age of four or five, sat down in front of a piano or a canvas or a chessboard and instantly became a concert pianist or a world-renowned artist or a chess master—he or she was instantly successful. Most of us expect that our weight-loss journey will be like that little genius who instantly, after one note, one brush stroke, or one chess move, was perfect at the craft.

Guess what? Not so. Most of us suck at most things before we get good at them. That is why Bernoulli's equation is so on target. The odds of us achieving things are a challenge because none of us are instantly good at anything—we have to work for it. Our weight loss in the past has been elusive and therefore the odds of it happening this time go up even further.

Here's my point: Stop being a statistic. The studies show that only 10 percent of people who lose a significant amount of weight will keep it off for longer than a year.[83] I know—what a terrible way for me to end our time together. The point is this: Stop calculating the odds and the stats. Sure, Bernoulli had a point. The value of what we want is directly dependent on how badly we want it and how hard it is to achieve. But remember: Health *has* value and therefore achieving it is worth the odds. If you confine your behaviours to just crunching the numbers you will continue to push that elusive change beyond the horizon. Instead, learn from yourself—learn from your mistakes and increase your potential.

I have tried in these pages to give you some teachings to help in the everyday. My last lesson is this: Start teaching yourself. You have by now figured out who you are with regards to your patterns of behaviour. Don't stop there. You have undoubtedly, throughout this book, gained some ideas about where to begin your own path to change. If that is not the case, then perhaps it was at least a pleasant read. But if you did learn something about what you are doing now and what you need to do in the future to be healthier in your approach to food and exercise, than I challenge you to go beyond the possibilities.

Weight loss is hard. Our genetics and our physiology fight it every step of the way. But to stop there is an insult to humanity. To suggest that disease is a state that we must accept is an offence to all of us who spend each day in the trenches searching for cures. My challenge to you is to take what you have learned in this book and confront your own genetics and your own physiology. Don't ever settle for what you have been given in life. I have learned all too well in medicine and in life that we take what we are given and we make the best of it. I've tried in my life and with my patients to do just that—now it is your turn. Go for it. I'll be cheering you on every step of the way.

Don't Go at It Alone

In 2010 Vancouver hosted the Winter Olympics (you may have heard about it). I was really lucky to be in the middle of it all. Like many Canadians we had a sense that we, as a nation, were really something. For sixteen days people cheered in the streets, literally. We went to restaurants, and regular diners would spontaneously break out into the national anthem and, of course, the remaining patrons chimed in. It was magical.

I sat at my first Olympic event, short-track speed skating, and watched something remarkable happen. First, let me say that speed skating fans are hard-core. I thought hockey fans were something, but apparently they have nothing on those who love short track. I watched as a packed stadium screamed at the top of their lungs for their given nation, and I couldn't help but wonder, *"What would life be like if we went to work every day and had a crowd cheering us on?"* Would I be a better doctor if every time I made the right diagnosis a crowd would appear at the bedside and applaud? Would my parents have been better teachers if after every great class their students stood up with signs and foam fingers and chanted their names?

And then I wondered, "*What about my patients?*" Could the same be said for their weight-loss success? Don't we all need a little cheering squad once in a while? Studies show that marathon runners do indeed run faster, even in the last few kilometres when they are otherwise physically spent, just by hearing the roar of a crowd.[84] What athlete doesn't look into the camera once in their career and talk about the importance of the fans in their victory? People need a fan base, and weight loss and healthy change is no different. I have always maintained that we get sick in silent, dark places. When we start to talk and listen in the light of day we give ourselves a chance to get well.

Margaret is fifty-four years old. She is easily sixty pounds overweight. She has decided to embark on a weight-loss journey to improve her health. She has told no one about her visit today, and she insists that none of her family find out what she is doing. "I need to do this on my own. I don't want anyone to know." She is adamant.

When we get to the scale, Margaret tells me that I can weigh her on one condition: "Don't tell me what the number is. I don't want to know." I explain to Margaret that although the scale is not the only tool we use for measuring weight loss, it is an important one for us to see how she is doing in her weight-loss pursuits. "I don't care. I don't want to know." Perhaps Margaret sees the scale as "the enemy." Perhaps if she does not know how much she weighs she does not have to face her weight problem head-on. Perhaps the number on the scale is a significant source of shame and she does not want those emotions to colour her world. Perhaps a million other reasons explain why Margaret does not want to know that number on the scale.

What Margaret has done with her actions thus far is to isolate herself—she has single-handedly done it *her way*, but her way is a lonely one. By cutting herself off from the reality of her current situation she has also limited her ability to know the truth and to be held accountable. Furthermore, Margaret has prohibited her family from being her very important cheering squad.

Studies show that people do indeed do better when they are accountable. A large-scale weight-loss trial took participants and randomized them into groups that either had one-on-one monthly contact with a physician or had self-accountability, meaning they just did things on their own. Here's a shocker—the group that checked in with someone regularly lost 20 percent more weight and kept it off for the length of the study compared to the do-it-yourself group.[85] Furthermore, studies show that accountability is most successful when it is accompanied by positive reinforcement and when people feel encouraged by their "coach."[86]

Here's the lesson from this example: Go in with your eyes wide open. Whether you are Margaret or not, find someone to check in with periodically throughout your weight-loss journey—a friend, your family doctor, a counsellor, a personal trainer, a nutritionist, and so on. We all need someone to be accountable to and, most importantly, someone who will cheer us on when we feel the weight of the world beating down on us.

Margaret's new plan is a secret to everyone around her. If she decides one day not to follow through, her world will be none the wiser. No one will check in to see how things are going. If she stops coming to her doctor's appointments it will be as if she never started anything. Furthermore, how can Margaret's world prepare itself for the changes she wants to make if she has not alerted the people in it?

So forget the silent treatment and forget trying to do this on your own. Here are some steps to make accountability a powerful positive force in your path to a healthy future:

1. **Keep your eyes wide open.** Know your starting point. Get on a scale, take your measurements, and know your blood pressure, cholesterol, and other metabolic numbers (like blood sugar and so on). Know what your risk is. If you know what you are dealing with you can prepare yourself for the road ahead.
2. **Find a plan.** Hopefully the previous chapters have given you a place to start. Maybe they have not and you've just found this to be an entertaining experience; if that is the case, put this book down immediately and start looking for something that meets your needs.
3. **Get yourself a coach.** We all need one person who is a sounding board of support to help us stay on track and guide us through the storms. You know who you can count on in this world—now go ask for their support.
4. **Get a cheering squad.** Inspiration comes in the strangest forms and from the most unlikely places. People around you will be amazingly supportive if they know that you are in search of a better way of life—just ask. If they refuse, then perhaps you might want to

re-evaluate a few relationships, but that's a decision I leave in your capable hands.

In addition to a team, there are certain tools that can be very helpful for accountability's sake:

Your Food Diary

A food diary in itself is one of the most useful tools in the accountability armament. Learn to use it wisely. As highlighted previously, there is evidence to support the use of a food diary in making behavioural changes, so try and find a way to make it work for you.

The Scale

A scale is only one part of the puzzle and should not be the only thing to keep you on track. It is a crude measurement in many respects. Remember that weight fluctuates based on time of day and time of month. It can also be easily affected by water retention, lack of sleep, and travel. Do not use the scale as your only guide, but it is a helpful tool. I recommend to patients to weigh themselves at home on a weekly basis. Make sure it is at the same time of day and get a decent bathroom scale. It does not have to be a clinical-grade scale like the one I have in my office, but it should be one that can weigh you accurately and is reasonably priced.

Remember not to let the number guide your behaviour too much, though. If you are up a pound or two it is not time for trash talk, and if you are down a few pounds it is not time for a party. Use the scale to reinforce what you already know and not to determine how you feel about yourself.

Margaret and I are working through her fears and her secrecy, and she has seen the power of asking for help and the rewards that it brings. Remember that when we isolate ourselves we deny others the opportunity to help us. Asking for help is one of the bravest things we can do, but also one of the most rewarding things. Ask for help from those around you and you will be amazed at how the world lines up to help. So be brave and let others help you—it is likely to be one of the smartest things you ever do.

15

A Plan of Action: Your Seven-Day Meal Plan

I know for some of you an actual blueprint for a better tomorrow may be just what you need to start you on your way to a healthier future, so here you go. I have put together a set of healthy meals to start you on your path of mindful eating. In each section you will find a list of better breakfasts, lunches, dinners, and snacks for you to "mix and match" to create your own meal planner.

Some of these meals are of my own creation and use the recipes found in the next chapter (these items are highlighted for you). I suggest you pick a few select meals to start with and use them in your everyday planning. This will allow for a more seamless transition than outlining a full seven-day meal plan. You can also adjust the meals to suit your specific tastes and dietary restrictions. Let's get started.

Breakfasts

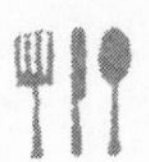

As I've already mentioned, breakfast really is an essential meal. The evidence shows that starting a day with food in your stomach is one of the key requirements for healthy living and weight reduction.

More importantly, what you eat to start the day can often set the tone for more mindful eating. Here is a list of seven healthy breakfast options with some tips on how to make them quick and convenient.

Breakfast 1

1 cup Oatmeal Magic with fresh fruit or berries (350 calories)

There are two ways to make oatmeal. The first is the old-fashioned way using quick oats or steel cut oats—this is my preferred method. I recommend you cook your oatmeal on a Sunday night and put about 1 cup into five different containers for the week. They can be refrigerated or even frozen and heated up every morning. This means you have old-fashioned, high-fibre oatmeal every morning without the labour-intensive process. Add some fresh fruit or berries and you have a nutritious, low-calorie meal. If you can't make oatmeal then stick with an instant variety that has no sugar added.

Breakfast 2

My Favourite Protein Bar and a piece of fruit (360 calories)

Protein bars can be very personal—everyone has a favourite brand and flavour. Stick with ones that are no more than 300 calories and have at least 10–20 grams of protein in them. These make a perfect fast and convenient breakfast on the go. If you are really ambitious you can use my recipe for homemade protein bars as well. They freeze well and can be made in advance.

Breakfast 3

Whole-wheat toast with peanut butter and banana (440 calories)

Make sure you stick with natural, no-sugar-added peanut butter. Measure out 2 tbsp at the most and add a sliced banana on top instead of jam. This gives you a healthier alternative to jam that is higher in fibre and low in added sugars.

Breakfast 4

Veggie Scramble (350 calories)

The recipe in the next chapter gives you several options for a veggie scramble, but you can also add your own choices to it. These can be made up to two nights before and simply heated up in the microwave in the morning.

Breakfast 5

Fruit with Greek yogurt (350 calories)

Greek yogurt is much higher in protein than regular yogurt and tends to fill you up more efficiently. Stick with about 1 cup of a low-fat variety (2% or less) and use about a cup of berries or chopped fruit. Add 2 tbsp of Superseed Mix and you have yourself a pretty nutritious meal. An easy variation on this is to replace the yogurt with low-fat cottage cheese.

Breakfast 6

Breakfast Protein Shake (300–400 calories depending on which one you choose)

There are a few recipes in the next chapter for a variety of different smoothie options. Easy and perfect for people who are trying to start to eat breakfasts.

Breakfast 7

Breakfast burrito (440 calories)

So easy to make. Take a small whole-wheat tortilla and add one scrambled egg, ¼ cup low-fat refried beans, and ¼ cup shredded cheese. Add some diced tomatoes and lettuce. Help yourself to some Hot Stuff Salsa and you have a pretty amazing way to start the day.

Lunches

Below I've given you seven midday meals that are convenient, nutritious, low calorie, and portable. You can mix and match to vary your meal plan as you wish. Remember that any of the International Salad recipes in the next chapter make a perfect lunch. Most of them can be made in "batch form" and will keep for almost the entire week. I usually make two or three for the week to get a great source of vegetables at lunch. You can easily add your own protein (chicken or a can of tuna) to them as you see fit.

Lunch 1
2 **Salmon Patties** (these really are amazing, and I am not biased in the least!) (250 calories)
Cut up veggies with 1/2 cup Low-Fat Dip (100 calories)
1 cup blueberries (70 calories)
420 calories total

Lunch 2
Village Greek Salad (320 calories)
1/2 pita with 1/2 cup hummus (200 calories)
Piece of fruit (70 calories)
590 calories total

Lunch 3
2 cups **Superfoods Salad** (300 calories)
Piece of fruit (70 calories)
370 calories total

Lunch 4
California Salad with 6 ounces grilled chicken (450 calories)
Piece of fruit (70 calories)
520 calories total

Lunch 5
4 cups **Middle Eastern Salad** (377 calories)
Piece of fruit (70 calories)
447 calories total

Lunch 6
Sandwich Wrap (396 calories)
2 cups of **Asian Slaw** (100 calories)
496 calories total

Lunch 7
Last night's leftovers—whatever was for dinner last night is what is for lunch today. This is perfect for smaller families or single cooks; you never have to worry about what to do with a little bit of leftovers!

Dinners

Whether it's a family affair or dinner for one, you don't have to compromise on taste for convenience and health. The dinner plans below give you options to make the meals your own. You can use the recipes from the next chapter as a guide or as gospel. Either way, I'm happy to share some of my favourite meals in the hopes that you and your family will love them for their taste and nutritious value. You will also see that each dinner is roughly no more than 500 calories per serving.

Dinner 1

2 cups **Chili** (300 calories)
Mixed greens salad with low-fat Italian dressing (80 calories)
Whole-wheat roll for dipping (150 calories)
530 calories total

Dinner 2

5 ounces grilled chicken breast with Apple Sauce Marinade (150 calories)
2 cups **Wild Rice Casserole** (300 calories)
Mixed greens salad with low-fat dressing (80 calories)
530 calories total

Dinner 3

5 cups **Buffalo Borscht** (300 calories)
Whole-wheat roll for dipping (150 calories)
450 calories total

Dinner 4

5 ounces grilled pork chop with Apple Sauce Marinade (200 calories)
2 cups **Wild Rice Casserole** (300 calories)
Curried Cauliflower (100 calories)
600 calories total

Dinner 5

Not Your Mother's Pasta (300 calories)
Romaine salad with 3 tbsp low-fat Caesar salad dressing (store bought, any kind) and 2 tbsp Parmesan cheese (150 calories)
450 calories total

Dinner 6

5 ounces grilled steak (250 calories)
2 cups **Roasted Beet Salad** (250 calories)
500 calories total

Dinner 7

6–8 ounces **Barbecued Salmon** (200 calories)
California Salad (290 calories)
490 calories total

For those of you looking for an exact seven-day meal plan, simply pick one meal from each category and create your own. This will give you some flexibility and variations along the way. Remember to allow yourself one night out for dinner with those you love if that is important to you.

16

Recipes for Success

Breakfast Recipes

Breakfast Protein Shakes

1 serving

Chocolate Banana

1 scoop chocolate-flavoured protein powder (I use Vega brand)

1/2 cup (125 mL) coconut water

1 cup (250 mL) almond milk

1 frozen banana

1 tbsp (15 mL) sugar-free natural peanut butter

4 ice cubes

1 packet of Splenda or Stevia

Place all items in a blender or food processor and blend until smooth.

Nutritional analysis | Calories = 388 | Fat = 12.4 g | Carbohydrate = 42.5 g | Protein = 34.3 g | Fibre = 8.3 g

Berry Banana

1 scoop berry-flavoured protein powder (I use Vega brand)
1/2 cup (125 mL) low-fat Greek yogurt
1 cup (250 mL) almond milk
1 frozen banana
1 cup frozen blueberries or strawberries
1 packet of Splenda or Stevia

Place all items in a blender or food processor and blend until smooth.

Nutritional analysis | Calories = 433 | Fat = 5 g | Carbohydrate = 64 g | Protein = 44 g | Fibre = 11 g

Mocha Latte

1 scoop chocolate-flavoured protein powder (I use Vega Sport performance protein)
1/2 cup (125 mL) cold coffee
1 cup (250 mL) chocolate-flavoured almond milk
1 tsp (5 mL) instant coffee
1/2 cup (125 mL) low-fat Greek yogurt
4 ice cubes
1 packet of Splenda or Stevia

Place all items in a blender or food processor and blend until smooth.

Nutritional analysis | Calories = 245 | Fat = 5.5 g | Carbohydrate = 15 g | Protein = 43 g | Fibre = 3 g

The Green Monster

1 scoop vanilla-flavoured protein powder (I use Vega Sport performance protein)
1 cup (250 mL) almond milk
1 tbsp (15 mL) sugar-free natural peanut butter or almond butter
1 frozen banana
2 cups (500 mL) chopped kale
1 packet of Splenda or Stevia

Place all items in a blender or food processor and blend until smooth—make sure there are no chunks!

Nutritional analysis | Calories = 433 | Fat = 13 g | Carbohydrate = 53.4 g | Protein = 35.4 g | Fibre = 11.6 g

Banana Colada

1 scoop vanilla-flavoured protein powder (I use Vega Sport performance protein)
3/4 cup (175 mL) almond milk
3/4 cup (175 mL) coconut water
1 cup (250 mL) frozen pineapple
1 tsp (5 mL) vanilla
1 frozen banana
1 packet of Splenda or Stevia

Place all items in a blender or food processor and blend until smooth.

TIP: Cut up a bunch of bananas and place them in the freezer for use later in the week. You can do this with any fruit, including pineapple and berries.

Nutritional analysis | Calories = 316 | Fat = 4.5 g | Carbohydrate = 46 g | Protein = 30 g | Fibre = 10 g

My Favourite Protein Bar

24 servings

1 cup (250 mL) chocolate-flavoured protein powder (I use Vega sport performance protein)
1 cup (250 mL) whole-wheat flour
1/2 cup (125 mL) coconut
1/2 cup (125 mL) cocoa powder
1/4 cup (50 mL) flax seed
1/4 cup (50 mL) chia seeds
1/4 cup (50 mL) hemp seeds
1/2 tsp (2 mL) kosher salt
4 extra-ripe bananas
1 12-ounce (340 g) package of silken tofu
1/2 cup (125 mL) agave syrup or 1/4 cup Splenda
2 large whole eggs, beaten
1/2 cup (150 mL) natural peanut butter
Non-fat cooking spray

Line the bottom of a 13 × 9–inch glass baking dish with parchment paper and lightly coat with cooking spray. Set aside.

Preheat the oven to 350°F (175°C).

In a large mixing bowl, combine the protein powder, whole-wheat flour, coconut, cocoa powder, flax seed, chia seeds, hemp seeds, and salt. Set aside.

Using a potato masher or a fork, mash the bananas in a separate bowl.

In a third mixing bowl, whisk the tofu until smooth. Add the agave syrup (or Splenda), eggs, and peanut butter, one at a time, and whisk to combine after each addition. Add the bananas and fold the mixture together. Add to dry mixture and mix together.

Spread evenly in the prepared baking dish and bake for 40 minutes. Remove from the oven and cool completely before cutting into squares. Store in an airtight container for up to a week.

Nutritional analysis (per bar) | Calories = 185 | Fat = 9.7 g | Carbohydrate = 15 g | Protein = 13.4 g | Fibre = 9.7 g

Oatmeal Magic

4 servings

1 cup (250 mL) steel cut oats
3 cups (750 mL) boiling water
3/4 cup (175 mL) low-fat buttermilk
1 tsp (5 mL) vanilla
1/4 tsp (1 mL) cinnamon
2 ripe bananas
Non-fat cooking spray

Spray a large saucepan with non-fat cooking spray and add the oats. Stir on high heat for 2–3 minutes to toast. Add the boiling water and reduce heat to a simmer. Keep at a low simmer for 25 minutes, without stirring.

Add buttermilk to the oatmeal. Stir gently to combine and cook for an additional 10 minutes.

Spoon into a serving bowl and top with sliced bananas and cinnamon. Sweeten to taste (preferably with low-calorie sweetener!). You can also add a tablespoon of Superseed Mix for extra crunch!

TIP: You can substitute almond milk, skim milk, or even soy milk for the buttermilk. Substitute blueberries or apples for the bananas for a different taste.

Nutritional analysis | Calories = 217 | Fat = 3.3 g | Carbohydrate = 44 g | Protein = 8.7 g | Fibre = 5.6 g

Superseed Mix

1/2 cup (125 mL) flax seeds
1/2 cup (125 mL) chia seeds
1/2 cup (125 mL) hemp seeds
1/2 cup (125 mL) sunflower seeds
1/4 cup (50 mL) sesame seeds

Mix all ingredients together.

TIP: Makes a great topping for yogurt or oatmeal in the morning!

Nutritional analysis (per tbsp) | Calories = 45 | Fat = 3.4 g | Carbohydrate = 2.5 g | Protein = 2.0 g | Fibre = 1.9 g

Veggie Scramble

2 servings

4 eggs
2 tsp (10 mL) water
1 red pepper, chopped
1/2 red onion, chopped
10 mushrooms, chopped
1/2 cup (125 mL) vegetable or chicken stock
2 cups (500 mL) spinach
1/2 cup (125 mL) salsa (homemade or store bought)
Salt and pepper to taste
Fresh herbs to taste (optional)
1/2 cup (125 mL) shredded cheese of your choice
Non-fat cooking spray

Crack the eggs and beat with water until mixture is uniform. Set aside.

Spray a large skillet with the non-fat cooking spray. Add the mushrooms, onion, and peppers. Sauté with vegetable or chicken stock until vegetables are soft and the stock has evaporated. Add the spinach. Cover for about 3–4 minutes until spinach is wilted. Add salsa and stir for about 3–4 minutes until most of the liquid has evaporated.

Add in egg mixture and stir until eggs are cooked and fluffy.

Sprinkle with shredded cheese and leave on heat for about 1 minute until melted.

TIP: You can substitute 3 egg whites for 1 egg for more volume with the same calories; I usually use 3 eggs and 3 egg whites. You can also substitute 1 cup (250 mL) of chopped soft tofu for the eggs if you like—it tastes amazing!

Nutritional analysis | Calories = 360 | Fat = 22 g | Carbohydrate = 13.2 g | Protein = 27.5 g | Fibre = 2.8 g

International Salads

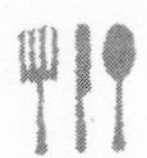

My patients always tell me they find eating the same salad one day after another *so boring* and they are always looking for ways to incorporate more vegetables into their diet. My solution is to think of salads as a trip around the world! Think of the vegetables native to a certain part of the world and you will have a great way to vary your salads and increase the amount of vegetables in your everyday diet. Here are my top international salads.

Asian Slaw

4 servings

1 package coleslaw mix OR 1 head each of red and green cabbage, shredded
1 cup (250 mL) carrots, shredded
1 red onion, very thinly sliced
1 cup (250 mL) frozen peas, thawed
1/2 cup (125 mL) sesame seeds

Dressing:
1/2 cup (125 mL) rice wine vinegar
2 tbsp (30 mL) sesame oil
2 tbsp (30 mL) soy sauce
2 tbsp (30 mL) honey

Optional Additions:

Shredded seaweed flakes and chopped pickled ginger to taste

Grilled chicken breast

Combine all ingredients for the dressing in a bottle or jar. Place the lid on the container and shake until smooth.

Place all vegetables in a container with a lid. Add dressing and shake until vegetables are covered.

Place in the fridge overnight.

TIP: This slaw is best eaten a day after it is made.

Nutritional analysis (per serving) | Calories = 208 | Fat = 11 g | Carbohydrate = 10.75 g | Protein = 5 g | Fibre = 8 g

California Salad

4 servings

1 bag of spring mix salad greens (about 8 cups/2 L)

2 cups (500 mL) of fresh strawberries, sliced

1 cup (250 mL) shredded carrots

1/2 cup (125 mL) goat cheese, crumbled

1/2 cup (125 mL) sliced almonds

Dressing:

1 cup (250 mL) red wine vinegar

3 tbsp (45 mL) olive oil

1/2 cup (125 mL) blackberries

Juice of 1 lemon

1 tbsp (15 mL) honey

2 cloves of garlic

Combine all ingredients for the dressing in a food processor and blend until smooth.

In a large bowl toss the salad greens, sliced strawberries, and shredded carrots.

Add dressing to taste until all vegetables are coated to your liking. Add goat cheese and sliced almonds.

TIP: You can keep the dressing on the side and then dip your fork into the dressing and then into the salad instead of pouring the dressing on the salad.

Nutritional analysis (per serving) | Calories = 291.5 | Fat = 18.5 g | Carbohydrate = 18.3 g | Protein = 11.5 g | Fibre = 5 g

Indian Chopped Salad

4 servings

2 English cucumbers
1 red onion
2 cups (500 mL) cauliflower
1 mango
1 can (19 oz/340 mL) chick peas (choose low-salt/no-salt-added variety), drained and rinsed
1 cup (250 mL) fresh mint, chopped

Dressing:
1/2 cup (125 mL) Greek yogurt
1/4 cup (50 mL) curry paste
2 tbsp (30 mL) olive oil
Juice of 2 lemons
Salt and pepper to taste

Dice all vegetables and the mango into small bite-sized pieces. Place into a large container with a lid.

Add chick peas and mint.

In a separate bowl, combine yogurt, curry paste, olive oil, and lemon juice. Whisk until smooth. Season to taste.

Add dressing to vegetables.

Place the lid on the container and shake.

TIP: You can use a food processor to finely chop vegetables and save yourself some work!

Nutritional analysis (per serving) | Calories = 295 | Fat = 14 g | Carbohydrate = 37.5 g | Protein = 8.5 g | Fibre = 8 g

Italian Chopped Salad

4 servings

1 head of romaine lettuce

1 jar (12 oz/355 mL) roasted red peppers packed in water, rinsed

1 can (14 oz/398 mL) artichokes, rinsed

3 roma tomatoes, chopped

1/2 red onion, chopped

10 green olives, sliced

10 black olives, sliced

1 can (19 oz/340 mL) white cannellini beans (you can use chick peas if you want)

1/3 cup chopped fresh basil

Optional proteins (per person):

1 grilled chicken breast, sliced

20 cooked shrimp, peeled

1 can of tuna, drained

Dressing:

1/2 cup (125 mL) balsamic vinegar

1/4 cup (50 mL) Dijon mustard

2 tbsp (30 mL) olive oil

Juice of 1 lemon

2 cloves of garlic, crushed

Salt and pepper to taste

Combine all ingredients for salad dressing in an empty bottle or sealed container and shake until smooth. Set aside.

Dice all vegetables into small bite-sized pieces. You can also use a food processor to save time. Place vegetables into a large container with a lid.

Add cannellini beans and basil. Add dressing to vegetables.

Place the lid on the container and shake.

Add optional proteins to top of salad, if desired.

Nutritional analysis (per serving, without optional proteins)
Calories = 286 | Fat = 12 g | Carbohydrate = 32.4 g | Protein = 7.5 g | Fibre = 8.5 g

Mexican Chopped Salad

4 servings

2 tbsp (30 mL) olive oil
2 cloves of garlic, minced
1 red onion, chopped
1 pound (454 g) lean ground beef or ground turkey or ground tofu substitute
1 cup (250 mL) salsa (homemade or store bought)
1 head of iceberg lettuce, shredded
3 tomatoes, chopped
1/2 cup (125 mL) olives, chopped
1 cup (250 mL) shredded cheese (any type of your choice)
Hot sauce to taste
1 cup (250 mL) low-fat sour cream
Non-fat cooking spray

Coat a skillet with non-fat cooking spray. Add olive oil, garlic, and red onion. Sauté until onion is soft.

Add ground beef or turkey or tofu and cook until brown.

Add salsa and combine. Remove from heat and let cool.

On a serving plate layer lettuce, tomatoes, olives, and cheese. Add meat/tofu mixture. Add hot sauce to taste and a dollop of sour cream.

TIP: You can also make this in a large, sealable container and keep in the fridge for later.

Nutritional analysis (per serving) | Calories = 550 | Fat = 6.75 g | Carbohydrate = 17.25 g | Protein = 44.25 g | Fibre = 3.75 g

Middle Eastern Salad

4 servings

1 cup (250 mL) Israeli couscous
2 tomatoes
2 English cucumbers
1 red onion
20 pitted kalamata olives
1 can (19 oz/340 mL) chick peas (choose low-salt/no-salt-added variety), drained and rinsed
1/3 cup (75 mL) balsamic vinegar
2 tbsp (30 mL) olive oil
Juice of 2 lemons
1 cup (250 mL) fresh mint, chopped
Salt and pepper to taste

Prepare Israeli couscous as per package directions and rinse with cool water.

Dice all vegetables into bite-sized pieces. Place into a large container with a lid.

Add chick peas, vinegar, olive oil, lemon juice, and mint.

Place lid on the container and shake.

TIP: You can use dried chick peas that have been soaked overnight and boiled, which will eliminate any added salt from canned chick peas. Substitute quinoa or kamut for the Israeli couscous.

Nutritional analysis (per serving) | Calories = 377 | Fat = 8.5 g | Carbohydrate = 61 g | Protein = 7 g | Fibre = 8.5 g

Village Greek Salad

4 servings

2 tomatoes

2 red peppers

1 English cucumber

1 red onion

1 cup (250 mL) feta cheese, cut into cubes or crumbled

20 pitted kalamata olives

1/3 cup (75 mL) balsamic vinegar

2 tbsp (30 mL) olive oil

Juice of 1 lemon

1 tsp (5 mL) oregano flakes

Pepper to taste

Chop all vegetables into bite-sized pieces. Place into a large container with a lid.

Add the feta cheese, olives, vinegar, olive oil, lemon juice, and spices. Place lid on the container and shake.

TIP: Add romaine lettuce to the Village Greek Salad for variation.

Nutritional analysis (per serving) | Calories = 326 | Fat = 21 g | Carbohydrate = 16.8 g | Protein = 12 g | Fibre = 3 g

West Coast Salad

4 servings

1 head of romaine lettuce, shredded

1 cup carrots, shredded

1 cup red onions, sliced

2 tomatoes, diced

1 large package of smoked salmon

1/4 cup (50 mL) capers

1/2 cup (125 mL) goat cheese, crumbled

Dressing:
1/2 cup (125 mL) balsamic vinegar
2 tbsp (30 mL) olive oil
2 tbsp (30 mL) maple syrup
Juice of 2 lemons
1 tbsp (15 mL) Dijon mustard

Combine all ingredients for the dressing in a bottle or jar. Place the lid on the container and shake until smooth.

Place all vegetables in a container with a lid. Add dressing and shake until vegetables are covered.

Add sliced smoked salmon, capers, and goat cheese.

Nutritional analysis (per serving) | Calories = 348.5 | Fat = 10.4 g | Carbohydrate = 19.1 g | Protein = 22 g | Fibre = 3 g

Lunch or Dinner Recipes

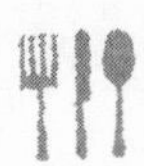

Barbecued Salmon

6 servings

1 whole salmon, head off, guts removed and cleaned OR 2 large salmon fillets
3 lemons, sliced
1 small jar of capers
1/2 red onion, thinly sliced
Salt and pepper to taste

Lay down one sheet of aluminum foil large enough to cover the fish.

If you are using a whole fish, place the whole salmon in the middle of the foil. Stuff the belly of the salmon with the sliced lemons, capers, and onions. Wrap in foil like a package.

If you are using 2 salmon fillets, lay one salmon fillet on the foil and cover it with sliced lemons, capers, and onions. Cover with the second fillet of salmon and wrap in foil.

Barbecue for about 15–20 minutes, depending on the size of the fish, until salmon is pink in the centre. Let sit for 5 minutes before unwrapping the foil.

Nutritional analysis (per serving) | Calories = 213 | Fat = 9 g | Carbohydrate = 1 g | Protein = 28.2 g | Fibre = 0 g

Buffalo Borscht

12 servings

2 tbsp (30 mL) olive oil
2 cloves of garlic, crushed
2 pounds (912 g) buffalo steak, cubed
2 cans (14 oz/398 mL) sliced beets with the juice
2 jars (500 mL) stewed purple cabbage
8 cups (2000 mL) vegetable or chicken stock
1 tsp (5 mL) Splenda
Salt and pepper to taste
Low-fat sour cream

In a large saucepan or soup pot, brown the garlic in the olive oil.

Add cubes of buffalo steak and brown.

Add beets (including the juice), cabbage, and vegetable/chicken stock.

Simmer on medium heat for about 2 hours, stirring periodically.

Add Splenda (I like my borscht a little sweet) and salt and pepper to taste.

Garnish with low-fat sour cream.

TIP: This soup freezes really well.
You can substitute a can of chick peas and a can of red kidney beans for the buffalo to make this a vegetarian soup.

If you don't like buffalo you can use lean beef, like a lean cut of flank steak.

Nutritional analysis (per serving) | Calories = 255 | Fat = 15 g | Carbohydrate = 6.4 g | Protein = 21.3 g | Fibre = 0.7 g

Chili

8 servings

2 tbsp (30 mL) olive oil
1 red onion, chopped
3 cloves of garlic, chopped
1 large can (19 oz/340 mL) chopped tomatoes, no salt added
1 large can (19 oz/340 mL) crushed tomatoes, no salt added
1 can (19 oz/340 mL) chick peas, no salt added
1 can (19 oz/340 mL) red kidney beans, no salt added
1 can (19 oz/340 mL) black beans, no salt added
1 cup (250 mL) edamame, shelled
1/2 cup (125 mL) chopped jalapenos (add more to taste)
1/2 cup (125 mL) hot sauce
2 tbsp (30 mL) chili powder
3 cups (750 mL) fresh spinach

Optional Additions:
1/2 cup (125 mL) white chia seeds (optional)
1/2 cup (125 mL) chopped cilantro (optional)
1 pound (454 g) lean ground beef or ground turkey, browned
2 cups (500 mL) firm tofu, chopped

In a large saucepan, brown the garlic and onions in the olive oil.

Add tomatoes, beans, edamame, jalapenos, hot sauce, chili powder, and cilantro. Slowly add spinach, stirring until it is reduced down.

Add chia seeds (if desired) and stir.

Simmer on low heat for about an hour, stirring periodically.

TIP: This freezes amazingly well.

Nutritional analysis (per serving, without beef, turkey, or tofu)
Calories = 200 | Fat = 5.5 g | Carbohydrate = 28.8 g | Protein = 11 g | Fibre = 8.5 g

Curried Cauliflower

4 servings

1 large cauliflower
2 tbsp (30 mL) curry paste
1 cup (250 mL) vegetable stock
1/2 cup (125 mL) low-fat coconut milk
1/2 cup (125 mL) chopped mango

Cut cauliflower in thin slices.

In a large saucepan, combine curry paste and vegetable stock and bring to a simmer.

Add cauliflower, coconut milk, and mango. Simmer on low heat until cauliflower is soft and well cooked.

TIP: You can use a package of frozen cauliflower that has been thawed in place of fresh cauliflower.

Nutritional analysis (per serving) | Calories = 104 | Fat = 5.5 g | Carbohydrate = 13 g | Protein = 1.5 g | Fibre = 2.6 g

Not Your Mother's Pasta Sauce

8 servings

Sauce:
2 tbsp (30 mL) olive oil
5 cloves of garlic, chopped
4 cups (1000 mL) mushrooms, sliced

6 cups (1500 mL) fresh spinach

6 tomatoes, cut into cubes

1 can (19 oz/540 mL) crushed tomatoes, no salt added

20 kalamata olives

1/2 cup (125 mL) vegetable stock

1 can (5 oz/156 mL) tomato paste

1/2 cup (125 mL) fresh basil, chopped

1/4 cup (50 mL) fresh oregano, chopped

1/4 cup (50 mL) fresh thyme, chopped

1 tsp (5 mL) pepper

1 cup (250 mL) low-fat ricotta cheese

Optional Additions:

1 pound (454 g) browned ground turkey

1 grilled chicken breast

In a large saucepan, sauté garlic in olive oil. An alternative is to use 1/4 cup (50 mL) of vegetable stock instead of the olive oil to sauté the garlic.

Add mushrooms and spinach and sauté until well done.

Mix in chopped and crushed tomatoes, olives, and vegetable stock and cover the pot. Simmer on low heat until the vegetables are well done and in a sauce consistency.

Stir in tomato paste.

Add fresh herbs and pepper and remove from heat.

Fold in ricotta cheese.

Nutritional analysis (per serving, without turkey) | Calories = 136.5 | Fat = 8.3 g | Carbohydrate = 10.8 g | Protein = 6.5 g | Fibre = 2.6 g

Nutritional analysis (per serving, with turkey) | Calories = 211.5 | Fat = 11.8 g | Carbohydrate = 10.8 g | Protein = 17.9 g | Fibre = 2.6 g

"Noodles"

4 servings

1 large spaghetti squash, cut in half and seeds removed
Olive oil in a spray bottle
Salt and pepper to taste

Preheat oven to 375°F (190°C).

Put each half of the spaghetti squash on a cookie sheet with the inside facing up.

Spray with olive oil from the spray bottle. Sprinkle with salt and pepper.

Bake for 40 minutes until the squash is tender and soft.

Remove squash from oven and let cool slightly. Using a spoon, scrape the squash from the skin and place in a serving bowl. Top with spaghetti sauce and serve with Parmesan cheese.

TIP: You can also use whole-wheat pasta instead of spaghetti squash for variation.
This dish makes great lunch leftovers!

Nutritional analysis (1 cup/250 mL) | Calories = 31 | Fat = 0.6 g | Carbohydrate = 7g | Protein = 0.6 g | Fibre = 0 g

Roasted Beet Salad

4 servings

3 raw red beets
3 raw golden beets
Olive oil in a spray bottle
Salt and pepper
1/4 cup (50 mL) balsamic vinegar
1/4 cup (50 mL) pine nuts
1/2 cup (125 mL) goat cheese, crumbled

Preheat oven to 375°F (190°C).

Peel and clean beets and cut into thin slices, then into quarters.

Place beets on a cookie sheet. Spray with olive oil from spray bottle and sprinkle with salt and pepper.

Bake for about 30–45 minutes until beets are tender.

Let beets cool. In a bowl combine beets, balsamic vinegar, and pine nuts.

Sprinkle with goat cheese and serve.

Nutritional analysis (per serving) | Calories = 238.5 | Fat = 16.5 g | Carbohydrate = 14.3 g | Protein = 10.3 g | Fibre = 6 g

Salmon Patties

20 servings

2 cans (7 oz/198 mL) pink salmon, drained
2 cans (7 oz/198 mL) sockeye salmon, drained
1 cup (250 mL) smoked salmon, chopped
1/2 cup (125 mL) frozen edamame, thawed
1/4 cup (50 mL) capers, drained and rinsed
1/4 cup (50 mL) barbecue sauce (you can substitute with chopped roasted red peppers)
4 eggs
1/2 cup (125 mL) flax seeds
1/3 cup (75 mL) whole-wheat bread crumbs
Non-fat cooking spray

Preheat oven to 375°F (190°C).

Place salmon in a bowl. Mash with a fork as you would if you were making salmon salad.

Chop smoked salmon into very small pieces and add to canned salmon.

Add edamame, capers, and barbecue sauce.

In a small bowl beat the eggs. Add to salmon mixture and combine.

Fold in flax seeds and bread crumbs.

Spray a cookie sheet with non-fat cooking spray.

Take salmon mixture and make small patties. Place them on the cookie sheet.

Bake for about 20 minutes until the bottoms are golden brown.

TIP: I use no-salt-added salmon, or you can use the leftovers from the Barbecued Salmon recipe!
These taste amazing cold the next day and will keep in the fridge for 3–4 days.

Nutritional analysis (per serving) | Calories = 105 | Fat = 5.4 g | Carbohydrate = 3.4 g | Protein = 9.7g | Fibre = 0 g

Sandwich Wrap

2 servings

2 small whole-wheat flour tortillas
2 tbsp (30 mL) Eggplant Dip
2 tbsp (30 mL) Hummus
4 oz (115 g) sliced turkey breast from the deli counter
1 jar (12 oz/355 mL) roasted red peppers, drained and rinsed
1 tomato, sliced
1 cup (250 mL) spring mix salad greens

Spread equal parts eggplant dip and hummus on the flour tortillas.

Add half of the turkey, red peppers, and sliced tomatoes to each tortilla.

Add a handful of spring mix salad greens to each tortilla and roll into a wrap.

TIP: You can substitute any kind of luncheon meat or even sliced grilled chicken or barbecued salmon for the turkey. You can also use cheese instead of meat or fish if you prefer.

Nutritional analysis (per serving) | Calories = 396 | Fat = 10.9 g | Carbohydrate = 36.5 g | Protein = 34 g | Fibre = 10.4 g

Superfoods Salad

12 servings

1 cup (250 mL) cooked black quinoa
1 cup (250 mL) cooked red quinoa
1 cup (250 mL) cooked kamut
6 cups (1500 mL) kale, chopped
1/2 cup (125 mL) fresh mint, chopped
20 pitted kalamata olives
1 red onion, chopped
3 cups (750 mL) Swiss chard, chopped
Seeds from 1 pomegranate OR 30 red grapes cut in half
1 can (19 oz/540 mL) chick peas, no salt added, drained and rinsed

Tahini Dressing:
3 tbsp (45 mL) olive oil
3 tbsp (45 mL) tahini paste
Juice of 3 lemons
1/2 cup (125 mL) red wine vinegar
1/2 cup (125 mL) water
1 clove of garlic, crushed

In a food processor, combine tahini dressing ingredients. Blend until smooth.

In a large sealable container combine all salad ingredients. Add dressing, and salt and pepper to taste.

Close lid and shake.

Nutritional analysis (per serving) | Calories = 214 | Fat = 7.7 g | Carbohydrate = 30.3 g | Protein = 6.8 g | Fibre = 4.5 g

Wild Rice Casserole

6 servings

1 cup (250 mL) wild rice
5 cups (1.25 L) fresh mushrooms, sliced

1 cup (250 mL) chick peas

3 cups (750 mL) vegetable stock

1 tsp (5 mL) salt

1 tsp (5 mL) pepper

3 cloves of garlic, chopped

1/4 cup (50 mL) chopped fresh sage

Soak wild rice in 5 cups (1.25 L) of water overnight. Drain and rinse the rice the following morning.

Preheat oven to 375°F (190°C).

In a casserole dish, mix all ingredients. Cover with a lid and bake for an hour.

Remove from the oven and stir. The liquid should be completely absorbed into the rice. If there is still some liquid left, put the dish back in the oven for about another 20 minutes.

TIP: I like to use a variety of mushrooms in this dish: morels, porcini, chanterelles, crimini, portobello, etc. You can use whatever mushrooms you like.

Nutritional analysis (per serving) | Calories = 186 | Fat = 1.3 g | Carbohydrate = 35 g | Protein = 7.7 g | Fibre = 7 g

Dips and Marinades

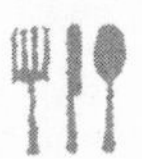

Apple Sauce Marinade

Makes about 1 cup (250 mL)

1/4 cup (50 mL) balsamic vinegar

1 cup (250 mL) unsweetened apple sauce

2 tsp (10 mL) Worchester sauce

2 cloves of garlic, chopped

Combine all ingredients in a bowl.

TIP: This is a perfect marinade for barbecue pork chops. Place pork chops in a container and spread marinade over the meat. Leave in the fridge in the morning and when you get home from work they are ready for grilling.
If time does not allow, you can put the marinade on pork chops and cook immediately.

Nutritional analysis (for the entire marinade, excluding pork)
Calories = 89 | Fat = 0 g | Carbohydrate = 20 g | Protein = 0 g |
Fibre = 1 g

Eggplant Dip

Makes about 3 cups (750 mL)

2 large eggplants, sliced
Olive oil in a spray bottle
Salt and pepper to taste
1/4 cup (50 mL) vegetable stock
2 tbsp (30 mL) tahini paste
1 tsp (5 mL) cumin

Preheat oven to 375°F (190°C).

Place slices of eggplant on a cookie sheet and spray with olive oil. Sprinkle with salt and pepper.

Bake for 30 minutes until eggplant is tender. Remove from the oven and allow to cool.

Place eggplant in a food processor with vegetable stock, tahini, and cumin. Blend on high until a paste forms.

TIP: Roasted mushrooms can be substituted for the eggplant for a variation on this dip.

Nutritional analysis (1/4 cup/50 mL) | Calories = 48 | Fat = 2.8 g | Carbohydrate = 5.8 g | Protein = 1.6 g | Fibre = 2.7 g

Hot Stuff Salsa

Makes about 2 cups (500 mL)

4 tomatoes, diced
1 red onion, diced
1 cup (250 mL) cilantro, chopped
1/2 cup (125 mL) jalapenos, chopped
1/4 cup (50 mL) red wine vinegar
1 tbsp (15 mL) olive oil

Combine all ingredients in a food processor or just chop all the vegetables finely and combine.

Nutritional analysis (1/2 cup/125 mL) | Calories = 47 | Fat = 3.4 g | Carbohydrate = 4.5 g | Protein = 0 g | Fibre = 2 g

Hummus

Makes about 1 cup (250 mL)

1 can (19 oz/540 mL) chick peas, no salt added, drained and rinsed
1/2 cup (125 mL) vegetable stock
1 tbsp (15 mL) olive oil
2 tbsp (30 mL) tahini paste
4 cloves of garlic, chopped
Salt and pepper to taste

Combine all ingredients in a food processor and blend on high speed until a smooth paste forms.

Nutritional analysis (2 tbsp/30 mL) | Calories = 75 | Fat = 3.8 g | Carbohydrate = 8.5 g | Protein = 2.5 g | Fibre = 2 g

Low-Fat Dip

Makes about 2½ cups (625 mL)

1 cup (250 mL) low-fat sour cream
1 cup (250 mL) fat-free mayonnaise
1 tbsp (15 mL) Dijon mustard
1 tbsp (15 mL) balsamic vinegar
1/4 cup (50 mL) fresh parsley, chopped
3 cloves of garlic, chopped
Salt and pepper to taste

Combine all ingredients in a food processor and blend on high speed until smooth.

Nutritional analysis (2 tbsp/30 mL) | Calories = 20 | Fat = 1 g | Carbohydrate = 2.2 g | Protein = 0.4 g | Fibre = 0.15 g

All-Fruit Sherbets

These sherbets are my healthy alternative to ice cream and a fun way to increase your fruit intake. They are best made right before eating. I serve them with fresh fruit as the perfect end to a meal. The key is to make sure the fruit used is frozen. A food processor is a must when making these.

Banana Colada Sherbet

4 servings

2 frozen bananas
2 cups (500 mL) frozen pineapple
1/2 cup (125 mL) coconut water

1/2 cup (125 mL) plain, unsweetened almond milk or skim milk
1 packet of artificial sweetener

Combine all ingredients in a food processor and blend on high speed until smooth.

Nutritional analysis (per serving) | Calories = 140 | Fat = 2 g | Carbohydrate = 33 g | Protein = 1 g | Fibre = 3.8 g

Mango Pineapple Sherbet

4 servings

2 cups (500 mL) frozen mango, chopped
2 cups (500 mL) frozen pineapple
1/2 cup (125 mL) coconut water
1/2 cup (125 mL) plain, unsweetened almond milk
1 packet of artificial sweetener

Combine all ingredients in a food processor and blend on high speed until smooth.

Nutritional analysis (per serving) | Calories = 133 | Fat = 1 g | Carbohydrate = 31.4 g | Protein = 0.5 g | Fibre = 3.8 g

Strawberry Lemon Sherbet

4 servings

2 cups (500 mL) frozen strawberries
Juice of two lemons
1/2 cup (125 mL) sugar-free pink lemonade
1 packet of artificial sweetener

Combine all ingredients in a food processor and blend on high speed until smooth.

Nutritional analysis (per serving) | Calories = 77 | Fat = 0.2 g | Carbohydrate = 20.2 g | Protein = 1 g | Fibre = 4.6 g

Afterword: Reflections on Lessons Learned

I'm often asked what I've learned from my professional and personal journey. Many of my colleagues wonder if significant weight loss can even be done through behavioural change alone. They ask if it is worth the massive effort working with people every day who struggle for what seems like an elusive goal. The days are long and the medicine is a challenge, that's for sure; there is no magic pill and I have both good days and bad. But I smile and think to myself, "This is just what I do; this is who I am." I'm not really sure that I would have been as satisfied with or as effective in any other field in medicine.

My friends wonder if my attitude toward food and exercise is really worth all the effort. Is it worth all the hard work and the days on a bike? Has the promise of better health been enough to keep the ice cream at bay?

At this point in life these questions seem irrelevant. Those who have made the transition to a healthier lifestyle will overwhelmingly tell you that yes, they do feel better and life is overall a better place. But more importantly, I have learned that people guard the status quo in life. We do what we do because we do it, and habits are just that—what we do. I am a doctor who practises a certain kind of medicine. I have seen the impact it has and I am a believer;

the science is there purely to back me up in my convictions. My everyday is really what confirms for me what I already know—it is *definitely* worth it.

As for the more personal question "Do you miss the ice cream?" I try not to think of it like that. You see, it's not about one door or another, or a life with or without. You don't say "goodbye" to ice cream and "hello" to health. I think that is a rather pedestrian attitude toward this whole process. Instead, I have learned that it is essential we understand that the fight to be healthy is an endless one and not a series of black-and-white choices. It's more about establishing a code of conduct that determines who you are, which affects every aspect of your life because it is *a part of you*. My patients teach me every day that the struggle makes the person more so than the result. The way we reach the healthier parts of ourselves, the way we work toward a better lifestyle really does determine who we are and what we are made of.

More than anything, though, I have learned that the end result, the mountains climbed and the things I can do now, are merely a sum of the struggle. If that is in fact the case, we should all welcome the battles to come—they are what will make us the people we strive to be tomorrow. You see, it's not about the ice cream left behind, it's about the challenges yet to be faced. Weight loss is hard. Health is not the default. Many of my colleagues would argue that significant long-term weight loss through diet and exercise is the exception and *not* the rule.

So what have I learned after all this time as both a patient and as an obesity doctor? It's quite simple: I've learned that we are all waiting to be exceptional—we just need an opportunity.

Notes

1. Schwart, M.W., Woods, S.C., Porte, D. Jr, Seely, R.J., & Baskin, D.G. (2000). Central nervous system control of food intake. *Nature, 404*, 661–671.
2. Albert, C.M. et al. (1998). Fish consumption and cardiac death. *Journal of the American Medical Association, 279*(1), 23–28; Albert, C. et al. (2002). Nut consumption and risk of cardiac death, physicians health study. *Archives of Internal Medicine, 162*(12), 1382–1387.
3. Gautier, J.F. et al. (2000). Differential brain responses to satiation in obese and lean men. *Diabetes 49*(5), 838–846.
4. Leibowitz, S.F., & Alexander, J.T. (1998). Hypothalamic serotonin control of eating behaviour, meal size and body weight. *Biological Psychiatry, 44*, 851–864; Di Marzo, V. et al. (2001). Leptin-regulated endocannabinoids are involved in maintaining food intake. *Mature, 410*, 822–825.
5. Drenowski, A. (1997). Taste preferences and food intake. *Annual review of Nutrition, 17*, 237–253.
6. Martinez-Hernandez, A. et al. (2006). Genetics of obesity. *Public Health Nutrition, 10*(10A), 1138–1144.
7. Stunkard, A.J. et al. (1986). A twin study of human obesity. *Journal of the American Medical Association, 256*(1), 51–54.
8. Frayling, T.M. et al. (2007). A common variant in FTO gene is associated with body mass index and predisposes to childhood and adult obesity. *Science, 316*, 889–894.
9. Cecil, J.E. et al. (2008). An obesity associated FTO gene variant and increase energy intake in children. *New England Journal of Medicine, 359*, 2558–2566.

10. Speakman, J.R. (2004). Obesity: The integrated roles of environment and genetics. *Journal of Nutrition, 134*(8), 20905–21055.
11. Gray D.S., & Fujioka K. (1991). Use of relative weight and body mass index for the determination of adiposity. *Journal of Clinical Epidemiology, 44*(6), 545–550.
12. Metropolitan Life Insurance Company. (1959). New weight standards for men and women. *Stat Bull Metropolitan Life Insurance Company, 40,* 1.
13. Keyes, A. et al. (1972). Indices of relative weight and obesity. *Journal of Chronic Disease, 25*(6–7), 329–343.
14. Berrington de Gonzalez, A. (2010). Body-mass index and mortality among 1.46 million white adults. *New England Journal of Medicine, 363*(23), 2211–2219.
15. Wang, Y. (2008). Child obesity and health. *International Encyclopedia of Public Health* (Cambridge, MA: Academic Press), 590–604.
16. Gale, E.A. (2002). The rise of childhood type 1 diabetes in the twentieth century. *Diabetes, 51,* 3353–3361.
17. Reaven, G.M., Bernstein, R., Davis, B., & Olefsky, J.M. (1976). Nonketotic diabetes mellitus: Insulin deficiency or insulin resistance? *American Journal of Medicine, 60,* 80–88.
18. Sims, E.A. et al. (1973). Endocrine and metabolic effects of experimental obesity in man. *Recent Program of Hormone Resistance, 29,* 457–496; Qatanani, M., & Lazar, M. (2007). Mechanism of obesity-associated insulin resistance: Many choices on the menu. *Genes and Development, 21,* 143–145.
19. Wells, K.B., Lewis, C.E., Leake, B., & Ware, J.E. Jr. (1984). Do physicians preach what they practice? A study of physicians' health habits and counseling practices. *Journal of the American Medical Association , 252,* 2846–2848.
20. Our rising ad dosage: It's not as oppressive as some think (2007, February 15). *Media Matters,* www.mediamatters.org/research.
21. Harris, J.L. et al. (2009). Priming effects of television food advertising on eating behaviour, *Health Psychology, 28*(4), 404–413.
22. Cummings, D.E. et al. (2002). Plasma ghrelin levels after diet-induced weight loss or gastric bypass surgery. *New England Journal of Medicine, 346,* 1623–1630; Hansen, T.K. et al. (2002). Weight loss increases circulating levels of ghrelin in human obesity. *Clinical Endocrinology, 56*(2), 203–206.
23. Mars, M., de Graaf, C., Van-Rossum, C., De-Groot, C., Seidell, J., & Kok, F. (2005). Leptin and appetite responses induced by a four-day energy restriction: Preliminary results. *Appetite, 39,* 247; Weigle, D.S., Cummings, D.E., Newby, P.D. et al. (2003). Roles of leptin and ghrelin in the loss of body weight caused by a low fat, high carbohydrate diet. *Journal of Clinical*

Endocrinology Metabolism, 88, 1577–1586; Chin-Chance, C., Polonsky, K.S., & Schoeller, D.A. Twenty-four-hour leptin levels respond to cumulative short-term energy imbalance and predict subsequent intake. *Journal of Clinical Endocrinology Metabolism, 85*, 2685–2692.

24. Morton, G.J. et al. (2006). Central nervous system control of food intake and body weight. *Nature, 443*(21), 289–295.
25. Hagan, M. et al. (1999). Role of the CNS melanocortin system in the response to overfeeding. *Journal of Neuroscience, 19*, 2362–2367.
26. Ahima, R.S. et al. (1996). Role of leptin in the neuroendocrine response to fasting. *Nature, 382*, 250–252.
27. Ahima, R.S. (2008). Revisiting leptin's role in obesity and weight loss. *Journal of Clinical Investigation, 118*, 2380–2383.
28. Enriori, P.J. et al. (2006). Leptin resistance and obesity. *Obesity, 14*, 254S–258S.
29. Zheng, H. (2007). Eating for pleasure or calories. *Current Opinion in Pharmacology*, 7(6), 607–612.
30. Zheng, H. et al. (2009). Appetite control and energy balance in the modern world: Reward driven brain overrides repletion signals. *International Journal of Obesity, 33*, S8–S13.
31. Ibid.
32. Adam, T.C. et al. (2007). Stress, eating and the reward system. *Physiology & Behaviour, 91*(4), 449–458.
33. Zentner, A. et al. (2010). Characteristics of obese patients presenting to community-based weight loss program. Abstract submitted to American Heart Association Annual Meeting.
34. Gearhardt, A.N. (2009). Preliminary validation of the Yale Food Addiction Scale. *Appetite, 52*(2), 430–436.
35. Johnson, R.J. et al. (2007). Potential role of sugar (fructose) in the epidemic of hypertension, obesity and the metabolic syndrome, diabetes, kidney disease, and cardiovascular disease. *American Journal of Clinical Nutrition, 86*, 899–906.
36. Jalal, D.I. et al. (2010). Increased fructose associated with elevated blood pressure. *Journal of the American Society of Nephrology, 21*, 1–7.
37. Dhingra, R., Sullivan, L. et al. (2007). Soft drink consumption and risk of developing cardiometabolic risk factors and the metabolic syndrome in middle-aged adults in the community. *Circulation, 116*, 480–488.
38. Nakagawa, N. et al. (2005). A causal role for uric acid in fructose induced metabolic syndrome. *American Journal of Physiology, 290*(3), 625–631.
39. Almiron-Roig, E. et al. (2003). Liquid calories and the failure of satiety: How good is the evidence? *Obesity Reviews, 4*(4), 201–212.
40. www.calorieking.com.

41. Schlosser, E. (2001). *Fast food nation: The dark side of the all-American meal* (New York, NY: First Mariner Books).
42. Canadian Community Health Survey. Available at www.hc-sc.gc.ca/fn-an/surveill/nutrition/commun/cchs_guide_escc-eng.php.
43. 2007 World Population Data Sheet on fast-food consumption.
44. Canadian Office of Consumer Affairs on restaurant and prepackaged food consumption.
45. Wansink, B. et al. (2005). Bottomless bowls: Why visual cues of portion size may influence intake. *Obesity Research, 13*(1), 93–100.
46. Rolls, B.J., Roe, L.S., Meengs, J.S., & Wall, D.E. (2004). Increasing the portion size of a sandwich increases energy intake. *Journal of the American Dietetic Association, 104,* 367–372.
47. Canadian Community Health Survey on household consumption, 1970–2004. (2007).
48. Young, L.R., & Nestle, M. (2002). The contribution of expanding portion sizes to the U.S. obesity epidemic. *American Journal of Public Health, 92*(2), 246–249; Nielsen, S.J., & Popkin, B.M. (2003). Patterns and trends in food portion sizes, 1977–1998. *Journal of the American Medical Association, 289*(4), 450–453; Smiciklas-Wright, H., Mitchell, D.C., Mickle, S.J., Goldman, J.D., & Cook, A. Foods commonly eaten in the United States, 1989–1991 and 1994–1996: Are portion sizes changing? *Journal of the American Dietetic Association, 103*(1), 41–47.
49. Wen, C.P. et al. (2011). Minimum amount of physical activity for reduced mortality and extended life expectancy: A prospective cohort study. *Lancet, 378*(9793), 741–848.
50. Manson, J.E. et al. (2002). Walking compared with vigorous exercise for the prevention of cardiovascular events in women: Data from the Women's Health Initiative Observation Study. *New England Journal of Medicine, 347,* 716–725.
51. Powell, K.E., Thompson, P.D., Caspersen, C.J., & Kendricks, J.S. (1987). Physical activity and the incidence of coronary artery disease. *Annual Review of Public Health, 8,* 253–287; Berlin, J.A., & Colditz, G.A. (1990). A meta-analysis of physical activity in the prevention of coronary heart disease. *American Journal of Epidemiology, 132,* 612–628.
52. Knowler, W.C., Barret-Connor, E., Fowler, S.E., et al. (2002). Reduction in the incidence of type 2 diabetes with lifestyle intervention or metformin. *New England Journal of Medicine, 346,* 393–403.

53. Chakravarthy, M. et al. (2003). Eating, exercise and "thrifty" genotypes: Connecting the dots toward an evolutionary understanding of modern chronic diseases. *Journal of Applied Physiology, 96*(1), 3–10.
54. Holloszy, J.O. (1976). Biochemical adaptations to endurance exercise in muscle. *Annual Review of Physiology, 38,* 273–291; Green, H.J. (1991). Early muscular and metabolic adaptations to prolonged exercise training in humans. *Journal of Applied Physiology, 70*(5), 2032–2038.
55. Gwinup, G. (1975). Effect of exercise alone on the weight of obese women. *Archives of Internal Medicine, 135,* 676–680; Oscai, L.B., & Williams, B.T. (1968). Effect of exercise on overweight middle-aged males. *Journal of American Geriatric Society, 16,* 794–797.
56. Miller, W.C. et al. (1997). A meta-analysis of the past 25 years in weight loss research using diet, exercise, and diet and exercise intervention. *International Journal of Obesity, 21,* 941–947; Garrow, J.S., et al. (1995). Meta-analysis of exercise with or without dieting on body composition of overweight subjects. *European Journal of Clinical Nutrition, 49*(1), 1–10.
57. Wing, R.R. (1999). Physical activity in the treatment of the adulthood overweight and obesity: Current evidence and research issues. *Medicine and Science in Sports and Exercise, 31*(suppl.), S547–S552.
58. King, N.A. et al. (1997). High dose exercise does not increase hunger or energy intake in free living males. *European Journal of Nutrition, 51,* 478–483; King, N.A. et al. (1995). Exercise-induced suppression of appetite: Effect on food intake and implications for energy balance. *European Journal of Clinical Nutrition, 48,* 715–724.
59. Kissileff, H.R. et al. (1990). Acute effect of exercise on food intake in obese and non-obese women. *American Journal of Clinical Nutrition, 52,* 240–245.
60. Cunningham, J.J. (1991). Body composition as a determinant of energy expenditure: A synthetic review and a proposed general prediction equation. *American Journal of Clinical Nutrition, 54*(6), 963–969.
61. Poehlman, E.T. et al. (1991). The impact of exercise and diet restriction on daily energy expenditure. *Sports Medicine, 11*(2), 78–101; Hunter, G.R. et al. (2008). Resistance training conserves fat-free mass and resting energy expenditure following weight loss. *Obesity, 16*(5), 1045–1051.
62. Garrow, J.S., & Summerbell, C.D. (1995). Meta-analysis: Effect of exercise with or without dieting on the body composition of overweight subjects. *European Journal of Clinical Nutrition, 49*(1), 1–10.
63. Hansen, T.K. et al. (2002). Weight loss increases circulating levels of ghrelin in human obesity. *Clinical Endocrinology, 56*(2), 203–206.

64. Cummings, D.E. (2003). Roles for ghrelin in the regulation of appetite and body weight. *Archive of Surgery, 138*(4), 389–396.
65. Sumithran, P. et al. (2011). Long-term persistence of hormonal adaptations to weight loss. *New England Journal of Medicine, 365*(17), 1597–1604.
66. Achor, S. (2010). *The Happiness Advantage: The Seven Principles of Positive Psychology that Fuel Success and Performance at Work.* (New York, NY: Crown Publishing Group).
67. Stunkard, A.J., Thorkild, I.A., & Sorenson, M.D. (1993). Obesity and socioeconomic status: A complex relation. *New England Journal of Medicine, 329,* 1036–1037.
68. Gortmaker, S.L., Must, A., Perrin, J.M., Sobol, A.M., & Dietz, W.H. (1993). Social and economic consequences of overweight in adolescence and young adulthood. *New England Journal of Medicine, 329,* 1008–1012; Zhao, G., et al. (2009). Depression and anxiety among US adults: Associations with body mass index. *International Journal of Obesity, 33*, 257–266; Dixon, J.B. et al. (2003). Depression in association with severe obesity, changes with weight loss. *Archives of Internal Medicine, 163*(17), 2058–2065.
69. Diener, E. et al. (2009). Subjective well-being: The science of happiness and life satisfaction. In C.R. Snyder & S.J. Lopez (Eds.), *The Oxford Handbook of Positive Psychology* (New York, NY: Oxford University Press).
70. Ibid.
71. Fabricatore, A.N. et al. (2009). Predictors of attrition and weight loss success: Results from a randomized controlled trial. *Behaviour Research and Therapy, 47*(8), 685–691.
72. Bailey, A.A. et al. (1941). Phantom limb. *Canadian Medical Association Journal, 45*(1), 37–42.
73. Hollis, J.F. (2008). Weight loss during the intensive intervention phase of the weight-loss maintenance trial. *American Journal of Preventative Medicine, 35*(3), 118–127.
74. Johnson, R.K. et al. (2007). Personal digital assistants are comparable to traditional diaries for dietary self-monitoring during a weight loss program. *Journal of Behavioural Medicine, 30*(2), 165–175.
75. Hu, F.B., Stampfer, M.J., Rimm, E.B. et al. (1999). A prospective study of egg consumption and cardiovascular disease in men and women. *Journal of the American Medical Association, 281,* 1387–1394.
76. CBC News. (2012, July 10). Restaurant lunches costing Canadians, survey says. www.cbc.ca/news/canada/story/2012/07/10/lunch-eat-out-survey.html; MCNG. (2012, July 14). How often are Canadians eating out? www.mcngmarketing.com/how-often-are-canadians-eating-out/#.

UCNGFJhUkuk; Hellmich, N. (2009, June 3). The real "fast-food nation"? Not U.S., survey says. *USA Today*. www.usatoday.com/news/health/weightloss/2009-06-03-fastfood_N.htm.

77. Stellar, E. (1954). The physiology of motivation. *Psychology Review, 61*, 5.
78. Wing, R.R. (2001). Successful weight loss maintenance. *Annual Review of Nutrition, 21*, 323–341.
79. Health Canada and CDC Data, 2006.
80. Hmelo-Silver, C. (2004). Problem-based learning: What and how do students learn? *Educational Psychology Review, 16*(3), 235–266.
81. Sadato, N. et al. (1996). Activation of the primary visual cortex by Braille reading in blind subjects. *Nature, 380*, 526–531.
82. Gilbert, D. (2006). *Stumbling upon Happiness* (New York, NY: Random House Publishing).
83. Hollis, J.F. (2008). Weight loss during the intensive intervention phase of the weight-loss maintenance trial. *American Journal of Preventative Medicine, 35*(3), 118–127; Wing, R.R. (2001). Successful weight loss maintenance. *Annual Review of Nutrition, 21*, 323–341; Wing, R.R., Data from the National Weight Loss registry.
84. Hollis, J.F. (2008). Weight loss during the intensive intervention phase of the weight-loss maintenance trial. *American Journal of Preventative Medicine, 35*(3), 118–127; Wing, R.R. (2001). Successful weight loss maintenance. *Annual Review of Nutrition, 21*, 323–341; Wing, R.R., Data from the National Weight Loss registry.
85. Prochaska, J.O. (1992). In search of how people change: Applications to addictive behaviors. *American Psychologist, 47*(9).

Acknowledgments

Much of my life's work thus far has gone into this book. I am forever grateful for the support and guidance of those around me who have made it a reality. Firstly, to my patients, past and present, who inspire me every day with their courage and their humanity. I hope they feel this book is a compassionate and informative reflection of their disease and their struggles. I am grateful that many of them placed their confidence in me to tell their stories and I hope that I have respected that trust.

I want to thank my fitness trainers, who have pushed me physically and supported me mentally towards achieving my healthy goals. Mike Veinot, in particular—you always make me look forward to the gym, despite its shortcomings.

To my CBC family, thank you for being the place where it all began and for giving me a platform to push a healthy agenda.

To Andrea Magyar at Penguin Books, who has been the voice of reason from the very beginning of this project. You have championed this from the beginning and I can not thank you enough for your wisdom and your respect for the integrity of this piece. Many thanks to Mary Ann Blair, Leanne Rancourt and Helen Smith for your skill and attention to detail on this book.

A debt of gratitude must be paid to my teachers and mentors over the years. It indeed takes a village to raise a doctor and I was definitely a challenging pupil. Many thanks to Dr. Harvey Rabin and Dr. David Lau in particular who helped me learn from the best.

Finally on a personal note, I want to thank my family. I'd like to think my Dad would have been really proud of this book. He and my mother raised me with an unthinkably grand sense of confidence and self and thus far it has served me well. I am so fortunate to have had him as such a strong influence in my life if only for the time that I did. Mom, I am so lucky to be your kid. Your sense of compassion for others is a lesson the world could use more of. You are such a great lady who taught me that hard work is something to be proud of. Thanks for always "talking me over the bridge."

To Katina, my soul sister and the best doctor I know. I love that you "get me" and that is no small feat. Ours is a friendship for the ages. Many thanks to Sandy, my big sister and partner in crime. Your praise and support are always just the perfect medicine.

Finally, to my husband Jason. There are no words, despite the fact we have exchanged so many. Thanks for being both a captain and a willing passenger on this adventure. It's amazing to be loved so much and so well by such an extraordinary person. It gives you the strength to do anything. You are the best part of my day.

Index

C

D

F

APRIL - AT ALI'S OFFICE.
STARTING WEIGHT 266.5 POUNDS
BOUGHT THE WEIGHT LOSS PRESCRIPTION
FOUND ALI'S AUTOGRAPH INSIDE ☺
GOT TRULY INSPIRED TO START LIVING LIKE
I WOULD HAVE TO FOR THE REST OF MY LIFE
IN THE EVENT I HAD ALREADY HAD THE
GASTRIC SLEEVE DONE.